YOUR CHILD

Expert advice on raising healthy children

by Drs Douglas Cohen,
Kim Oates & John Yu
of the Royal Alexandra Hospital
for Children, Sydney

BayBooks
An imprint of HarperCollins*Publishers*

A Bay Books Publication

Bay Books, an imprint of
HarperCollins*Publishers*
25 Ryde Road, Pymble NSW 2073, Australia
31 View Road, Glenfield, Auckland 10, New Zealand

Revised edition first published in Australia by Bay Books in 1994
First edition published as *Care for your Child* by Bay Books in 1979

Text Copyright © Douglas Cohen, Kim Oates, John Yu 1994

This book is copyright.
Apart from any fair dealing for the purposes of private study, research, criticism or review, as permitted under the Copyright Act, no part may be reproduced by any process without written permission. Inquiries should be addressed to the publishers.

National Library of Australia
Cataloguing-in-Publication data:

Cohen, Douglas.
 Your child: expert advice on raising healthy children.
 New ed.
 Includes index.
 ISBN 1 86378 134 X

 1. Child rearing. 2. Children - Health and hygiene. I. Cohen, Douglas. Care for your child. II. Oates, R. Kim (Ronald Kim). III. Yu, John. IV. Title. V. Title: Care for Your Child.

649.1

Front Cover photo from The Photo Library
Internal illustrations by Karen Carter.
Printed in Australia by Griffin Press, Adelaide.

5 4 3 2 1
98 97 96 95 94

The publisher has made every effort to ensure that all contact details were correct when this book went to print.

About the Authors

DOUGLAS COHEN, AM, MB, MS, FRACS

Dr Cohen graduated in 1942 and, after War service with the AIF, spent ten years in general practice. In 1950 he obtained his senior degrees in Surgery and was appointed to the Children's Hospital.

During 1954–55 he worked in London, obtaining further experience in paediatric surgery, particularly in the newly developing field of cardio-thoracic surgery.

His interest in child safety resulted in the formation of the Child Safety Centre. He was the first Chairman of the Child Accident Prevention Foundation in NSW.

In 1971 he was appointed Head of the newly created Department of Paediatric Surgery at the Children's Hospital.

He is Past-President of the Australian College of Paediatrics and of the Pacific Association of Paediatric Surgeons.

He has been awarded Honorary Life Membership of the British, Australian and Canadian Associations of Paediatric Surgeons, the Australian College of Paediatrics and the Australian and New Zealand Cardiac Society.

In 1981 he was created a Member in the Order of Australia for his services to medicine, especially in paediatrics. He retired from clinical practice in 1988 and is currently living in London.

KIM OATES, MD, MHP, FRACP, FRCP, FRACMA, FAFPHM, DCH (RCP&S)

Dr Oates is Professor of Paediatrics and Child Health at the University of Sydney and Chairman of the Division of Medicine at the Camperdown Children's Hospital.

A graduate of the University of Sydney, he trained at the Children's Hospital at Camperdown, St Mary's Hospital in London and Boston Children's Hospital, returning in 1974 to head up Australia's first Community Paediatric Unit at the Children's Hospital. In 1985 he was appointed as the first Douglas Burrows Professor of Paediatrics and Child Health at Sydney University.

His main professional interests are general child health problems, child development, the prevention of child abuse and the care of developmentally disabled children. He is involved in medical research and education in Australia and overseas, being on the Board of the New Zealand National Child Health Research Foundation, a visiting Professor at the University of Colorado, USA and Professor of Paediatrics at Kunming Medical School, China.

The Board Chairman of the National Association for the Prevention of Child Abuse and Neglect in Australia and formerly President of the International Society for the Prevention of Child Abuse and Neglect, he has authored or edited eight books and published numerous scientific papers on a range of child health problems.

JOHN YU, AM, MB, FRACP, FRACMA, DCH (RCP&S)

Dr Yu graduated in Medicine from the University of Sydney in 1959 and joined the Resident Staff of the Royal Alexandra Hospital for Children in 1961. He studied at the Nuffield Neonatal Research Unit at Hammersmith Hospital 1963–1964 and returned to the Children's Hospital at the end of 1964. After two years of research at the University of Sydney, he was appointed to the Institute of Child Health and to the Honorary Medical Staff of the Hospital. He was appointed Head of the Department of Medicine in 1972, Deputy General Medical Superintendent in 1976 and General Superintendent and Chief Executive Officer in 1978.

He has served on the Councils of the Australian Paediatric Association, the Royal Australasian College of Physicians and the Australian Hospitals Association. He is a Trustee of the Malcolm Sargent Cancer Fund for Children and the Starlight Foundation.

He is interested in the arts and is an Honorary Associate of the Powerhouse Museum and a member of the Board of Trustees of that Museum. He has published widely in the decorative arts as well as in the field of medicine.

PREFACE

To 'care for' is defined in the *Concise Oxford Dictionary* as 'to feel concern or interest for, to provide food or attendance for, or to feel regard or affection for'.

Caring for children means all this and much more. It requires patience, understanding, honesty, a sense of humour and an indefinable ability to communicate that children recognise immediately. It can be tedious, time-consuming, repetitive and exacting. There are situations which would try the temper of the Archangel Gabriel himself. It involves the responsibility for decisions that can have far reaching consequences.

However, to see children grow and flourish in mind and body brings a deep sense of satisfaction, and to earn the trust and affection of a child is a reward beyond measure.

And that is the reason for this book: children are very important people.

In the following pages we have chosen to use the masculine and feminine genders in alternate chapters except where that is patently absurd.

We have also chosen to retain in this second edition the Foreword written by the late Emeritus Professor Sir Lorimer Dods in 1979. We do so to honour him as a great teacher and as one of the early advocates for children.

CONTENTS

ABOUT THE AUTHORS 3
PREFACE 5
ACKNOWLEDGEMENTS 10
FOREWORD 11

CHAPTER 1
CHILD CARE — WHAT THIS BOOK IS ABOUT 13

CHAPTER 2
SO YOU'RE HAVING A BABY 16
Development of the Baby 17
Chromosomes and Genes 18
Twins 19
The Newborn Baby 19
Loving Your Baby 22
Where Do Fathers Fit In? 22
Brothers and Sisters 22
Grandparents 23
Progress During The First Month 24
Babies Are Not Always Fun 25

CHAPTER 3
THE NEW ARRIVAL 26
Care of Your New Baby 26
Bath Time 27
Clothes for Baby 28
Infant Feeding 28
Breast-feeding
Breast-feeding at home
Formula-feeding
Facts and fables about breast-feeding
Feeding schedules
Some feeding difficulties
Weaning
Starting solids
Food Suggestions 35
Some first foods babies like
Meals for toddlers
Meals for kindergarten and school children
Fat Children and Thin Children 38
Fat children — what can we do?
Weight reducing hints for mealtimes
Some general hints
Mealtime Battles 41

CHAPTER 4
MILESTONES 42
Height and Weight 42
Seeing and Hearing 43
Speaking 43
Bilingual families 44
Social and Emotional Development 44
Bladder and Bowel Control 47
Teeth 47
Feet 49
Immunisation 49
Diphtheria, pertussis (whooping cough) and tetanus
Poliomyelitis (polio)
Measles, mumps and rubella (German measles)
Haemophilus influenza type B (HIB)
Hepatitis B
Immunisation schedule
Travelling with Children 52

CHAPTER 5
GROWING UP 54

Early Relationships Between
Mother and Baby *54*
Relating to Others *55*
Separation *56*
Death in the Family *56*
Baby-sitters *57*
Common Behaviour Problems *58*
Thumb sucking
Dummies
Comforters
Other comforting habits
Infantile colic
Sleep disturbances
Wakefulness in toddlers
Temper tantrums
Head banging and breath holding
Pica
Bad language
Jealousy and rivalry
Speech problems
Tongue tie
Stuttering
Nail biting
Sexual awareness
Bed-wetting

CHAPTER 6
CHILDREN AND PLAY 68

Play Material *68*
Play and Social Development *70*
Playing with Other Children *70*
Books and Stories *71*
Television *71*
Pets *71*
Suggestions for Play and Toys
at Different Ages *72*
The first year
Birth to six months

Six to twelve months
One to two years
Two to four years
Reading List *73*
For toddlers
Books to read to toddlers
For children four to seven
For children of all ages
Books about Australia
Play and the Sick Child *75*
Play and the Handicapped Child *76*

CHAPTER 7
HANDICAPPED CHILDREN 78

Physical Handicaps *79*
Deafness
Blindness
Delayed Development *81*
Down's syndrome
Management of developmental disability

CHAPTER 8
THE SICK CHILD 84

When to Call a Doctor *84*
Medicines *85*
Fever *85*
Problems of the Ears, Nose and Throat *85*
Coughs and colds
Croup
Nose bleeds
Sore throats, tonsillitis and swollen glands
Tonsils and adenoids
Middle ear infections (otitis media)
Glue ear
Outer ear infections (otitis externa)
Wax in the ears
Common Eye Problems *88*

Squint (strabismus)
Visual problems
Watering and discharging eyes
Conjunctivitis and styes
Itchy eyes
Eye injuries
Common Skin Problems *90*
Skin problems of infancy
Skin problems in older children
Bones and Joints *95*
Growing pains
Arthritis
Club foot (talipes)
Knock-knees and bow legs
Flat feet
Congenital dislocation of the hip
Scoliosis
Common Infectious Diseases *98*
Measles
Rubella (German measles)
Mumps
Whooping cough
Chicken pox
Roseola
Chest Problems *101*
Bronchitis and pneumonia
Asthma
Cystic fibrosis
Intestinal Problems *103*
Stomach aches
Constipation
Vomiting
Diarrhoea and vomiting — gastroenteritis
Appendicitis
Worms
Kidney and Bladder Problems *107*
Infections of the bladder and kidneys
Nephritis
Genital Disorders *108*

Vaginal discharge
Circumcision
Hernia and hydrocele
Undescended testis
Malignant Disease *110*
Congenital Malformations *111*
Congenital heart disease
Malformations of the bowel, kidney and lungs
Cleft lip and cleft palate
Spina bifida
Hydrocephalus
Some Other Childhood Illnesses *115*
Febrile convulsions
Allergies
Failure to thrive
Meningitis
Epilepsy
Diabetes
The Sudden Infant Death Syndrome (SIDS) *120*

CHAPTER 9
GOING TO HOSPITAL 121
Preparation for Hospital *121*
Preparation by play
Answering questions
Explaining facts
Pre-admission visiting
What to Take to Hospital *123*
What Happens After Admission *125*
Living In and Visiting *125*
Operations and Anaesthetics *126*
Day-stay Surgery *127*
Colds and Skin Rashes *127*
Loose Teeth *128*
Physiotherapy *128*
Going Home *129*

CHAPTER 10
CHILD SAFETY — HOW SAFE IS YOUR CHILD? *130*

Falls *131*
Cuts *131*
Burns and Scalds *131*
Poisons *131*
Inhaled and Ingested Foreign Bodies *132*
Electrical Safety *132*
Safety in the Backyard *132*
Water Safety *133*
Sunburn and Heat Exhaustion *134*
Barbecues and Incinerators *134*
Guns *135*
Pedestrian Safety *135*
Bicycle Safety *135*
Road Safety *136*
What To Do in an Emergency *137*
General
Cuts and falls
Burns and scalds
Poisons

CHAPTER 11
SOME SPECIAL FAMILY SITUATIONS *138*

Separation and Divorce *138*
Single Parents *139*
Step Families *139*
Working Parents *141*
Adoption *142*

CHAPTER 12
A LOOK INTO THE FUTURE *144*

Health Needs During Adolescence *144*
Puberty *145*
Puberty in girls
Puberty in boys
Pimples and spots
Adolescent Sexuality *147*
What is sexuality?
Sexual behaviour in teenagers *147*
Some of the harmful consequences
How can we help adolescents cope with their sexuality?
Some important facts teenagers should know
Juvenile Delinquency *151*
Drug Use by Adolescents *152*
Prevention
Signs of drug use
Normal Adolescent Behaviour *153*

SPECIAL INFORMATION FOR EMERGENCIES *155*

Choking *156*
External Cardiac Massage *156*
Mouth-to-mouth Resuscitation *157*

INDEX *158*

AKNOWLEDGEMENTS

The contributors to the first edition of this book were all experts in their own special fields. The majority of them are also experienced fathers and mothers — a few are grandparents as well! It was not feasible to ask them all to revise their original contribution so we take full responsibility for any changes to the text of this second edition.

Many colleagues contributed to the first edition of *Your Child* and their work is gratefully acknowledged. They included:

Bruce Benjamin, David Bennett, Sue Bissaker, Sue Creak, Genevieve Cummins, Michael Deloughery, Charles Enfield, Jim Friend, Keith Godfrey, Cynthia Gregory-Roberts, Wallace Grigor, Gabrielle Joshua, Ramanand Kamath, Julian Katz, John Keneally, Tony Lipson, Frank Martin, Hugh Martin, Craig Mellis, Archie Middleton, Margaret Mullaney, John Overton, Pamela Roberts, Suzanne Robertson, Paul Roy and Helen Walsh.

We are also grateful to Mrs Caroline Alexander for allowing us to quote from her very expressive letter about her profoundly deaf daughter, Megan.

Foreword

'With so much being written and said about child care today, many good parents have lost confidence in their parenting ability. All of us are different and your baby will also have his own characteristics, his own likes and dislikes. There can be no rules for good child care, just guidelines and commonsense.'

So begins the first chapter of *Your Child*. These most significant and reassuring words characterise the theme running through this excellent manual of commonsense child care which provides sound practical advice combined with repeated reassurance which is such an important component of happy and successful parenting. This reassurance begins in an early chapter with comforting words for the mother who cannot or does not wish to breast feed her baby, and continues through each section of this particularly helpful publication which abounds in easily understood definitions and explanations of many everyday problems in infancy, childhood and early adolescence.

It is my privilege to congratulate the authors, Mr Douglas Cohen, Dr Kim Oates and Dr John Yu, and their collaborators, who have happily and bravely accepted the special challenge of planning and writing this excellent book. I feel sure it will be of great practical value to parents of today and tomorrow.

Lorimer Dods

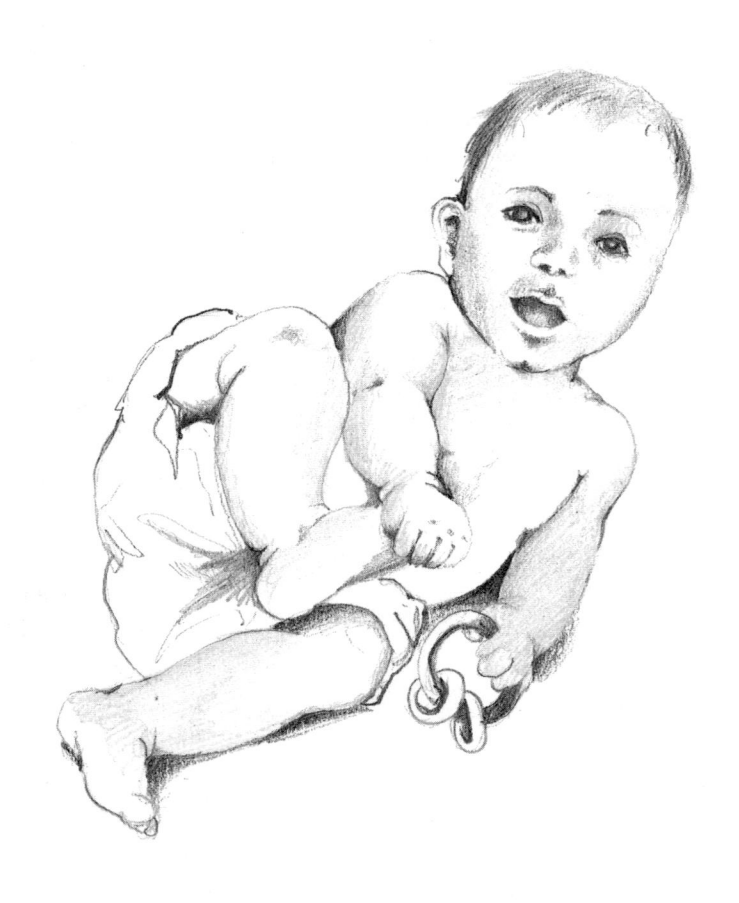

CHAPTER 1

CHILD CARE—WHAT THIS BOOK IS ABOUT

With so much being written and spoken about child care today, many good parents have lost confidence in their parenting ability. All of us are different and your baby will also have his own characteristics, his own likes and dislikes. There can be no rules for good child care, just guidelines and commonsense.

We hope that after you have read this book you will feel more confident to use your own commonsense and to bring up your child in a way best suited to you and your family. With this confidence, we are sure you will enjoy your baby and, by so doing, lay the foundations for a normal and happy childhood.

The physical needs of children vary according to their age. When they are babies, you will need to protect them from the extremes of weather, to keep them clean and to regularly provide them with food. With increasing age, most children can cope very much better with the environment and with less regular meals. There may even be times when they are too busy to eat!

The most important needs of children are to be loved and wanted. These needs may result in jealousies about brothers, sisters and even their own mother or father. This can be difficult to handle, especially when one child is ill and needs extra care and attention. Involving the other children in his care often helps them not to feel neglected and less loved.

Every child growing up presents conflicts between wanting to be mothered and wanting to be independent and grown up. If you understand this conflict you will be able to deal with your child's apparently opposing and inconsistent behaviour without becoming angry.

Parents often cannot understand why one of their children reacts in a particular way when the other children in the family who experience the same problems seem to cope without trouble. This depends on

It is important to allow children to talk about things that are bothering them
▼▼▼

the personality of each child and what particular strengths and sensitivities each one possesses. Such a variation is normal within both families and whole communities.

Later in childhood, there is a very strong need to belong and to feel that one belongs. Families are important but so too are friends, the youth group and the school. It's not easy to be different from the other children at school; an awareness of a child's anxieties in this regard and an understanding of her feelings may prevent a lot of unhappiness, even problems like school refusal, recurrent abdominal pains, leg pains and headaches. It is important to allow the child to talk about these things even though it may make you feel angry, embarrassed or even guilty. Ganging up on kids and calling them names is part of normal childhood behaviour: it does not have to be intentionally cruel, although the results of these actions may be very harmful to a child who does not feel secure within herself. Very often it is the bully who needs help.

The need to be loved and wanted may cause anxieties when both parents are working or away from home at the same time. What is important here is the nature and quality of the parent–child relationship when the family is together. Most children have more sense than we give them credit for; try telling them what is happening or needs to be done and don't worry if they don't seem to understand every word or concept. They will understand enough to be reassured.

The children of recently arrived families present their own special problems, particularly if the family does not speak English fluently or if there are racial characteristics, such as skin colour or customs which make them different from the majority of the people in the community in which they live. Many efforts are being made to minimise the problems these families face and in some hospitals, for example, there are full-time interpreters available to help. The interpreters are also very important as they help the staff to understand the differing attitudes and feelings migrant families may have about sickness, handicaps and death.

Most countries have different customs and ways of bringing up children and while they are undoubtedly very suitable for their own country, some of these methods may not be suitable for Australian conditions. A good example of this is the way many people from the Middle East swaddle their young very heavily and keep them from sunlight. This custom was important in their home country where the sun was very hot and bright, but in the temperate climate of Australia it may result in rickets.

Many standard Australian health practices, like

immunisation, are not freely available in less developed countries and so some new arrivals don't understand why immunisation is so important in keeping children healthy. If you are a new arrival, ask your family doctor, health centre or a children's hospital about the health programs that are available. There is usually literature printed in different languages about immunisation and other health programs. If you know newly arrived families with young children, help them to take advantage of our health programs by explaining to them about immunisation, family planning, and so on, or tell them where to get help.

It's particularly difficult when some children seem to reject all the customs of their homeland once in their new country and they may even seem to be ashamed of their own people, language and customs. This is almost always a transient or passing phase and results from the need of children, particularly in adolescence, to be like the group, not to be different. It's easy to understand why parents get angry, but if you try to understand how your child feels you will not only be able to minimise the hurt you feel yourself, but will also be able to help your child adapt and accept the good things about being different.

Our Aboriginal children present their own special problems which can vary depending on whether they come from the city, from country towns or from more remote areas. These problems are a complicated mixture of medical, cultural, social, economic, financial and environmental issues. There are governmental and special community organisations available to help with the management and care of these children, but only in recent years have we begun to understand how much damage the colonisation of Australia did to the health and culture of this country's original inhabitants.

Children need to feel they are part of a group
▼▼▼

Child care... 15

CHAPTER 2
SO YOU'RE HAVING A BABY

Caring for your child commences before baby arrives. Most parents have had no special training for what is one of the most important events in their lives. A good time for both parents to learn baby care is before baby's birth.

The first important decision is your choice of doctor and hospital. Try to choose a doctor in whom you feel you will have confidence, who will have the time and patience to answer your questions and who, you feel, will understand and support both you and your partner. Your family doctor may deliver your baby, or you may choose an obstetrician or a midwife.

Most maternity hospitals and birthing units conduct classes which both mothers and fathers are welcome to attend. In addition, it is usually possible for the mother-to-be to undertake exercises designed to make labour easier and to learn how to relax.

You are probably aware that some women develop a craving for particular foods during pregnancy and that others may become more emotional or more easily upset than usual. It's also common for many mothers to experience fears about their developing baby; whether it will be normal at birth and particularly whether they do anything that can harm the baby they are carrying. This applies especially to any medicines they may be taking, any illness during pregnancy and continuing intercourse after they are pregnant. It's best to discuss any such fears and anxieties with your doctor. Although pregnancy is a time of joy and fulfilment, it is also a time when such anxieties can emerge. After baby is born it's not uncommon for mothers to feel depressed, although there may be no obvious reason for this. If this feeling of depression continues or starts to interfere with your day-to-day life, you must seek your doctor's advice. Simple treatment is often available.

As pregnancy continues you will tend to become more and more preoccupied with thoughts and preparations for your unborn baby; the 'real world' around you may seem less important at this time.

DEVELOPMENT OF THE BABY

Conception or fertilisation occurs at the outer end of the Fallopian tube where the sperm unites with the ovum or egg. The ovum is about the size of the head of a pin, while the sperm is much smaller. The fertilised ovum passes on into the uterus (womb), where it attaches itself firmly to the wall. This area of attachment will become the placenta or afterbirth through which the developing baby obtains food and oxygen. All this time the fertilised ovum is continuing to divide and grow. The developing baby is attached to the placenta by the umbilical cord which contains the blood vessels which carry oxygen and essential foodstuffs from the placenta to the baby. The baby floats in fluid called the amniotic fluid, contained within a membranous sac attached to the edge of the placenta.

During the first eight weeks of pregnancy, the fertilised ovum divides rapidly and the various groups of cells that are formed differentiate into numerous

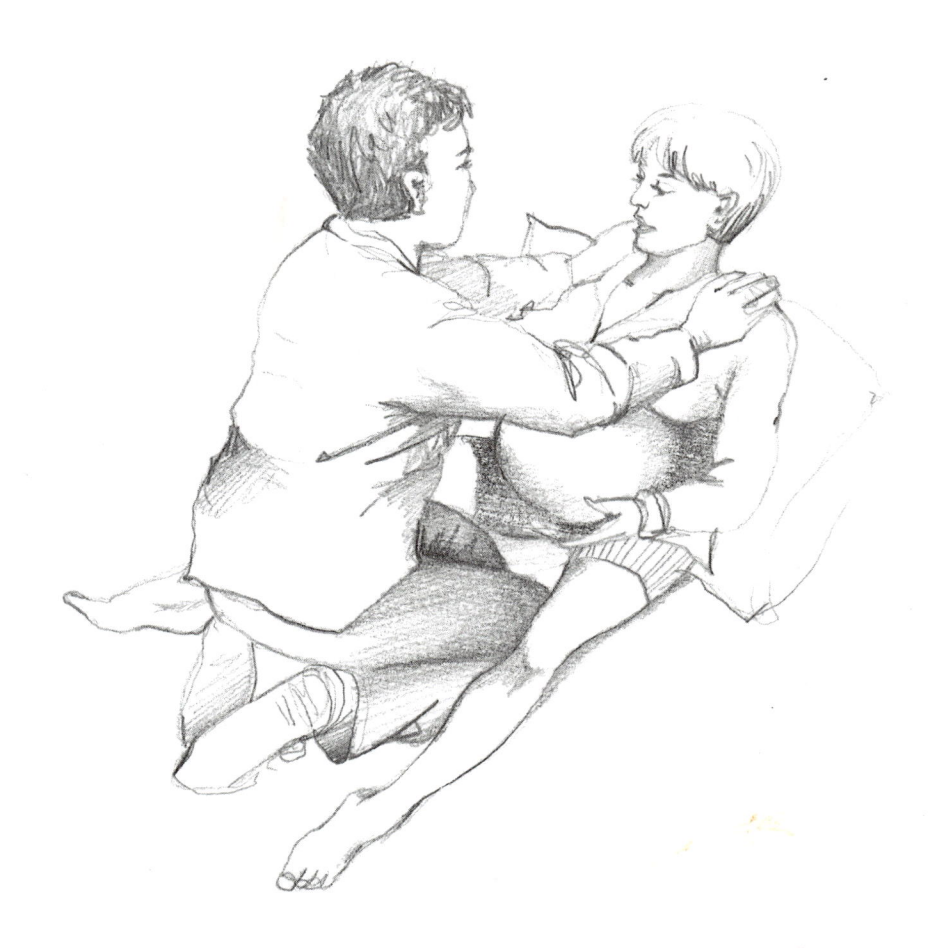

So you're having a baby

organs such as the brain, liver, lungs, eyes and heart. Small limb buds develop which will later form the arms and legs. By eight weeks, the developing baby or embryo is approximately 3 cm long and already has a tiny head and face, limb buds and the beginnings of all its internal organs. By twelve weeks, it is 8 cm long, the heart is beating and the kidneys and liver have started to work.

These first twelve weeks are a time of very rapid growth, and during this period all the baby's organs are formed and begin to function. This is the time at which damage to the baby can most readily occur. Certain drugs can damage the baby at this stage and this is the period when diseases contracted by the mother, such as German measles (rubella) and other viruses, have their most serious effects.

During the next three months rapid growth continues and baby's movements, which begin between sixteen and twenty weeks, become more active. All the vital organs are continuing to grow and are becoming progressively more mature. However, the vital organs are not sufficiently mature to maintain life should the baby be born at this early stage. By the end of the sixth month, baby is about 25 cm long and weighs around 800 g.

In the final three months of pregnancy, baby is preparing for her independent existence. She starts to deposit fat under the skin, builds up a store of glucose in her liver, and her bones become firmer. At the end of nine months, when she is fully mature, she weighs approximately 3.5 kg and is 52 cm long.

CHROMOSOMES AND GENES

Each cell of the developing baby carries forty-six chromosomes: twenty-three from the mother's ovum and twenty-three from the father's sperm. Along the chromosomes, like knots on pieces of wool, are the genes. These genes determine what we are like, including particular characteristics such as the colour of our eyes and hair and our facial appearance. Certain inherited diseases such as cleft lip and cleft palate and cystic fibrosis are transmitted by abnormal genes or an absence of genes. The science of genetics is now well established, and when parents have a child born with a malformation it is often possible to advise them about the chances of a similar malformation occurring in a subsequent pregnancy. It may also be possible to give advice to brothers, sisters and other close relatives about the chances of a similar problem affecting them or their children.

By twelve weeks, it is 8 cm long, the heart is beating and the kidneys and liver have started to work
▼▼▼

TWINS

Multiple births are rare but of these twins are the most common; your chance of having twins is about one in ninety, but it's greater if there are twins in the family already.

Twins can be identical or dissimilar. In identical twins both babies come from the same fertilised ovum and usually have a single placenta, though each baby has her own umbilical cord and bag of waters.

Dissimilar twins are completely different and come from two separate ova or cells which are shed from the ovaries and fertilised during the same menstrual cycle.

Twins are often born prematurely and, as the birth has a higher risk of complication, they should be managed in the larger obstetric units which have full paediatric facilities.

Mothers of twins face many additional domestic problems and challenges which can often only be met by a greater involvement of the father in day-to-day chores.

There are frequently worries about how to bring up twins, particularly identical twins, and the need to help them develop personalities of their own. It is not possible to generalise, but twins should be encouraged to develop their own interests and not be forced to behave and dress alike. If, however, they have common interests, it's wrong to force them to change just so they'll be different.

THE NEWBORN BABY

The newborn baby may look rather blotchy at birth and during the first few days of life. Her head is large in relation to her body and there is a gap, known as the anterior fontanelle, at the top of the skull. This is formed because the various bones that make up the skull have not yet fully fused together. It is covered by skin, and beneath that is a tough lining over the brain so that, although there is a boneless space, the underlying brain is really quite well protected and safe. The size of the fontanelle varies from baby to baby. The age at which the fontanelle closes is also quite variable and can range from about six months up to eighteen months.

At birth, the head may be an odd shape because it has had to mould to fit through the birth canal. The eyes may be bloodshot and there may be red marks on the eyelids or the back of the neck. These all eventually disappear and are not a cause for alarm. The baby will be covered at birth with a thick, greasy white material known as vernix designed to protect her skin in the womb and to make it easier

Slight jaundice in the first few days is common ▼▼▼

The baby will be covered at birth with a thick, greasy white material known as vernix ▼▼▼

for her to slip through the birth canal. Her body may be covered with fine hair which disappears over the first few weeks. Within a few days the head moulding and the skin marks disappear. You can often see tiny white spots on the face, looking like tiny pearls under the skin. These spots, called milia, are due to secretions that normally occur in the sweat glands. They disappear within a month or two and do not cause any problems.

During the last months before birth, the baby gets a good covering of fat. Premature babies miss out on this and so look small and thin at birth. They need special care to keep them warm in their early days and may take several months to make up their weight.

The breasts of newborn babies, boys as well as girls, are sometimes enlarged for the first few days of life. This temporary increase in size is caused by hormones crossing from the mother into the baby before birth. The breasts may even produce a few drops of milk. Don't worry, they will slowly get smaller. No treatment is necessary.

The stools of the baby are dark green and sticky for the first couple of days. This substance, known as meconium, gives way to the normal bowel actions. The range of normality for baby's motions is very wide. Breast-fed babies may have seven or eight soft, green stools each day, while other babies, particularly those on bottle feeds, may have less frequent brown-yellow formed stools, sometimes only on alternate days.

Some babies develop a brownish crust, often called cradle cap, on the top of the scalp. This is from a greasy substance the scalp produces and can be quite difficult to dislodge with ordinary washing. Gentle rubbing of baby oil or even olive oil into the scalp is often effective; allow it to soak in for five minutes before washing it off.

Sometimes you will see white blisters on the centre of the baby's lips. These are caused by sucking. Occasionally the skin peels on these blisters but they are painless, clear up by themselves and do not require any treatment. Slight jaundice in the first few days is common. It is caused by several factors, including the breakdown of the extra red blood cells which the baby needed before birth and by immaturity of the baby's liver.

The skin of a new baby is so soft, smooth and delicate that it is prone to a variety of rashes and blotches. Skin rashes, particularly on the face, are common in the first few weeks of life — so common that they can almost be classed as normal. Sometimes they are referred to as heat rashes or milk rashes, but usually the cause is unknown. It's tempting to change the brand of milk or even to stop breast-feeding in case the milk is not agreeing with the baby. This is almost never the case. Skin rashes and spots usually pass whether the milk is changed or not. As most commercial milks are very similar to each other, it is usually best to stick to the one you are familiar with and on which the baby is thriving.

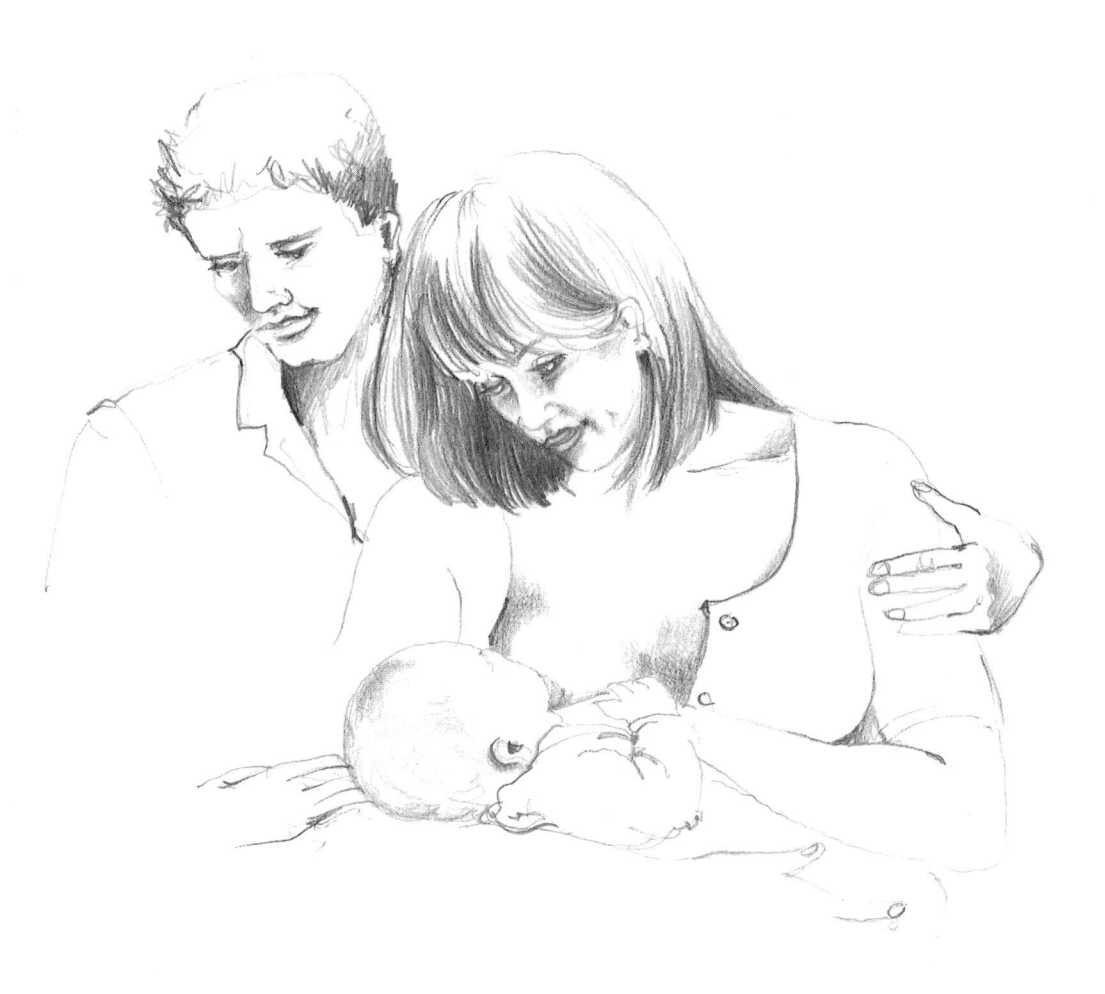

Even the best cared-for babies develop nappy rashes. These are usually caused by ammonia which is liberated from the baby's urine. Changing the nappies regularly reduces the amount of time baby's bottom is in contact with wet or dirty nappies. Nappy rashes can usually be kept to a minimum if the nappies are washed in a gentle soap product and well rinsed, if the nappy is changed frequently and if the baby is not kept in plastic pants for long periods. If a rash does start to appear, protect the red area with vaseline or a waterproof cream and let her lie exposed in the sun for short periods without a nappy so that the water logged skin can dry out.

LOVING YOUR BABY

A baby should be in her mother's arms as soon as possible after birth so that bonding can take place. Ideally, this should start at the moment of birth. Babies are very sensitive to their mother's care right from the beginning, so it's important to enhance this relationship in whatever way possible.

However, it's also important to understand that not all mothers are elated at the time of their baby's birth. Many are just tired and relieved that it is over. Many feel unsure about things at this stage — particularly new mothers who wonder if they really will be able to manage to look after their baby and to come to love her as much as everyone expects them to. It is usual to have worries like these. It is not unusual to be disappointed by your baby's appearance at first, to be disappointed with the sex or to worry that there is something wrong. For many, it takes time to fall in love with a baby and to feel confident about caring for her. This period of uncertainty is normal for many mothers.

During pregnancy, both mother and father usually have some preconceived ideas of what their baby will be like. This is usually an idealised picture and very often the baby you get is different from the baby you expect.

Babies are very sensitive to their mother's care right from the beginning
▼▼▼

WHERE DO FATHERS FIT IN?

For a father, having a baby is almost as important an event as it is for a mother, and he should have the opportunity of sharing this experience with his partner as fully as possible. Mothers need the support and love of their partners at this very important period in their lives together.

Hopefully, father will be involved during the pregnancy, perhaps attending some of the antenatal classes and attending the birth. It generally takes fathers a little longer than mothers to fall in love with their baby, although the more he is involved with the pregnancy the sooner this is likely to happen and the less he is likely to feel left out. The father's involvement in the care of his baby is vital for father – baby bonding. Fortunately, attitudes have changed and male society no longer ridicules fathers who become involved in some of the chores, as well as the fun involved in helping to care for the new baby.

BROTHERS AND SISTERS

If there are older brothers and sisters, they should be prepared for the new baby well before the

Your Child

birth. It helps if they can be involved in some small way in helping to prepare for the baby's arrival, perhaps by helping to sort out some baby clothes or having a small gift of their own to give the baby. The situation of a new baby coming home to stay can be rather threatening to a child, particularly if he had been the baby of the house until then.

It is quite normal for siblings to express feelings of anxiety or anger at this time. This is not only due to feelings of rivalry or jealousy about the new arrival but also to the unavoidable separation from their mother that takes place while she is in hospital for the birth of the new baby. Brothers and sisters can express their anxiety in a number of different ways. Sometimes they may be frankly aggressive and tend to pinch or hit the new baby. On the other hand, some children may repress their feelings and, as a result have nightmares or other sleep disturbances. Others may express their anxiety by reverting to more infantile behaviour. They often demand more attention, especially at feeding time when they want to climb up and sit on their mother's lap, too. Pushing them away or becoming angry with them just convinces them that their fears of being displaced by this newcomer are justified. Try sitting them near you on the floor and telling them a story while you feed baby. The situation can often be helped by giving them some sense of responsibility in helping to care for the baby.

Some parents arrange for their other children to be given a gift when the baby arrives and say that the gift is a present to them from the baby. The new little intruder is much more acceptable to her brothers and sisters if she arrives bearing gifts. But despite this, the new baby is still likely to be poked and pulled by his brothers and sisters who are curious about her and seek a reaction. It is important to realise that the new baby's presence might be quite worrying to them and parents should try to provide them with some extra care and time soon after coming home.

GRANDPARENTS

In the ideal situation, grandparents can gain great pleasure from their grandchildren and at the same time be a considerable help and support to young parents. But unfortunately, this happy state of affairs does not always exist as tensions are not uncommon when the new baby arrives home. Many young parents, having recently achieved independence, quite understandably don't wish to put themselves back in a dependent position. Also, some young mothers are sensitive about their inexperience and resentful of any criticism.

Most grandparents understand

Involve older siblings in helping to care for the baby
▼▼▼

Grandparents can provide much needed support to the new mother ▼▼▼

this and try hard not to interfere. On the other hand, they do have experience and judgement and may find it difficult not to express their opinion, particularly about things that have changed since they brought up their babies. A harmonious relationship, particularly between grandmother and new mother, requires tact and understanding on both sides. Nevertheless, there are so many advantages and so much happiness to be gained for all concerned that it is well worth the effort.

Grandparents can provide much needed support to the new mother. If, however, your family is not available to you, you should try to identify, well in advance, people who you feel can be helpful and supportive at this time, such as special friends, or possibly your family doctor or your church or religious centre.

Progress during the first month

During the first month your baby makes a great deal of progress, although at first it is not always obvious. Over the first few days her posture slowly changes from a curled-up position, as she was in the womb, into the more usual stretched-out position. She starts to learn to move her arms up and down, although it will be another four or five months before she is able to reach out and grasp objects. She may open and close her hands, but often keeps her fists gently closed during the first month. When placed on her back she will kick her legs alternately. The head is still quite floppy during this period although her neck muscles are becoming stronger. You will find that when she is placed face-down she can lift her head up for a few seconds and may turn her head from one side to the other.

A number of interesting reflexes can be observed at this time. Among these are the rooting and sucking reflexes which are essential for survival (see Chapter 3, Breast-feeding). When a finger is placed in the palm of her hand baby will unconsciously grasp it in a reflex fashion. This 'grasp reflex' is strong in the first few weeks and persists in a weaker form for about three months. It is not until this reflex is lost that the baby can learn to consciously grasp objects. The 'startle reflex' can be seen when the baby is suddenly startled or jolted. She throws her arms out on either side of her, opens her hands and may cry.

During the first month much of a baby's time is spent sleeping, crying or feeding. At the same time, she is constantly being bombarded with new and interesting sounds, sights, smells and sensations from her surroundings. It is a time for absorbing as much of this information as possible. These experiences are stored in her brain as she slowly builds up a picture of the world and its inhabitants. She is particularly responsive to a human face and seems to be able to find the eyes of the person looking at her and to fix onto them. Towards the end of the first month she is often beginning to smile back in response to her mother's or father's face.

All the cooing and gurgling that baby engenders is important from the very beginning. Talk to her softly and gently at every opportunity. At one or two months she will smile back and by four or five months she will laugh and gurgle in response. She is producing 'language' and you are helping her.

There is such a wide range in the 'normal' baby that, although many books describe the average baby, not many people have a baby quite like this. Some are at the very quiet end of the normal range, sleep for long periods, suck slowly and are fairly placid. Others are just the opposite, seeming to need even less sleep than their parents, feeding vigorously, wriggling constantly and crying with great fury at times. These two types of babies, as well as all those in between these two extremes, are normal babies who are starting to develop their own personality patterns and individuality even from this early stage.

BABIES ARE NOT ALWAYS FUN

Some aspects of caring for baby may be just plain drudgery. When it has been raining for three days and the house is hung with wet washing, when baby is letting you know in no uncertain terms that she is ready for dinner, when the telephone is ringing, the milk boils over on the stove, the dog is chewing baby's rattle and Grandma pops in for a surprise visit you may wonder if it is all really worth it. That is normal but fortunately, all this is more than compensated for by other times when you are able to play with her, talk to her and expose her to a variety of interesting stimuli to help her build up her picture of the world. It's good for her to hear different sounds and to feel different shapes and textures. It's very important for her to be talked to frequently. It will be a long time before she is able to talk back, but she will respond in other ways. Meanwhile, she will be storing away in her brain all the sounds and tones she hears in preparation for when she does start to talk.

Talk to your new baby softly and gently at every opportunity
▼▼▼

So you're having a baby

CHAPTER 3

THE NEW ARRIVAL

CARE OF YOUR NEW BABY

When you come home from hospital with your new baby, it's as if you are making a fresh start, not only for the baby, but for you and your family as well. This new baby is your main concern, but caring for him can be both trying and tiring if you are not prepared physically and emotionally for the task ahead.

It's important to remember that no two babies are alike. It's impossible to say to anyone: 'Here are ten rules, now follow them'. Each individual child has his own needs which are best judged by you. Finding out about these needs and responding to them will be a learning process for both baby and parents and one which will go on for many years.

Don't be worried about making decisions for your child's well-being, because there are many people who are able to help you. Your Baby Health Centre and your family doctor are both good sources of advice. A children's hospital is another good source of advice and one which is as close as the nearest telephone, twenty-four hours a day. Mothercraft support groups and Nursing Mothers Associations exist in most states and can provide a lot of help and support.

Although there are no strict rules about your baby's care, it is sensible to develop some routine and order at home and in your life to enable you to spend more time with your baby. This time spent with a new baby is important in forming the strong ties which will last a lifetime.

Initially your baby's needs are fairly basic: his feeding schedule is dictated by his tummy, but his bath time should be at a time to suit you. Try to speed up household chores and keep them to a minimum so you can spend time cuddling and talking to your baby. Don't let housework get you down, or take up too much of your time. Family and friends should be encouraged to make their own cup of tea while you nurse the baby! Organise your daytime hours. You have a job to do that won't fit into a day unless you are organised and set some priorities.

In these last few months you've probably taken more notice of television advertisements featuring babies being cared for by glamorous, organised mothers, and feel that this is how you should be twenty-four hours of the day. You can splash on some lipstick to brighten yourself up, but motherhood is comfortable; loving and caring, not about your tidy house or whiter than white washing, it is about your baby.

Parents have a few precious years ahead of them. Spend these years well and enjoy your baby.

BATH TIME

It's a good idea to bath baby before a feed so that he can have a good sleep afterwards. Bathing is necessary not only for a fresh, clean baby but also to allow you to handle him and to stimulate him.

Here are a few tips to make bathing baby more fun and less frightening for a new parent:

- Use a lightweight plastic bathtub on a table top or bench.
- Have two towels — one for wrapping and drying and one to lie him on.
- Have two washers — one for the face and one for the body.
- Use any reliable brand of bland baby soap, don't use scented ones.
- As baby gets bigger, be prepared for some splashing. A plastic apron is handy, but a towel, pinned around your neck, is softer for baby. Fill baby's bath with a handy jug or container. If you have a hose connection, well and good. Don't fill the bath at the tap and then try to lift it. Remember to always put the cold water in first, then put in the hot. This will prevent hot water scalds.
- Test the bath temperature with your elbow. The water should feel warm, not hot.
- Prepare everything before you pick baby up. It saves time and accidents.
- Never leave baby alone on the bench or table or turn away from him. It takes only a second for him to roll off.
- Always talk to baby while you are undressing him and washing him. You can indulge in as much cooing and gooing as you like. Baby enjoys hearing your voice and feeling you handle him. But don't leave him too long in the bath as babies lose heat rather rapidly and get cold. Make sure the room is adequately heated in winter.
- Don't be frightened to wash baby's head thoroughly. You can't hurt him. There is a soft area not covered by bone in the front of the skull but it is thoroughly protected by a firm, fibrous membrane.

After baby is bathed, dried and dressed, you can put him in his pram, which you should have made up before his bath. Or if you have friends with you, this is the time for them to have a cuddle while you do other things. A pram will also give you a chance to air his crib or cot mattress and blankets.

Indulge in as much cooing and gooing as you like
▼▼▼

CLOTHES FOR BABY

Most stores where baby goods are sold carry a list of what you will need. Start preparing early so that you won't have to hurry at the end of your pregnancy when you are feeling tired. Getting ready early also means that if baby is born prematurely you will be ready.

The number of articles you need will differ and the materials you choose will vary to suit the climate where you live. Here is a list of the basic garments your baby will need:

- Three or four cotton singlets
- Three or four wool or wool mixture singlets
- Four pairs of bootees for the first months, then socks
- Two or three woollen cardigans
- Two or three flannelette rugs and cotton rugs
- Three or four jumpsuits
- One or two outfits for special occasions
- Bibs
- Six pairs of plastic or protective pants to cover nappies
- Three dozen nappies, if you are not using a laundry service.

A nappy service saves a lot of time and trouble but you will still need a dozen nappies for emergencies. Various brands of nappy fasteners are now available if you prefer not to use nappy pins. Disposable nappies are often used but present disposal problems. Even if you use cotton nappies, some disposable ones are important for emergencies or when you are going out. Only use plastic overpants when going out, as they can be irritating if used all the time and predispose to nappy rash.

INFANT FEEDING

There are many ways to successful breast-feeding and each mother needs to choose the one most suitable for herself and her infant and which best fits the way the family lives. Doctors, nurses and dietitians, can advise parents and watch the infant's progress, but the aim is to produce a contented, healthy child who grows and develops normally. The special relationships that an infant develops with people, especially mother, are at first largely dependent on satisfactory feeding and the accompanying love and attention.

BREAST-FEEDING

Human milk is the most suitable food for most infants and normally contains every necessary nutrient. It also contains natural substances which protect against infection and does not cause allergy. Sudden unexplained deaths are less common in breast-fed infants and the emotional bond between the mother and her breast-fed

The special relationships an infant develops are largely dependent on satisfactory feeding and the accompanying love and attention
▼▼▼

infant is usually very close, although this is certainly not exclusive to breast-fed babies. Breast-feeding is desired by most mothers, but some are reluctant and may even actively wish to avoid it. Others, for domestic reasons or the need to go out to work, prefer bottle-feeding and there are some medical conditions affecting mothers or infants that make breast-feeding inadvisable. Women who do not breast-feed their infants should not feel guilty or in any way less of a mother.

Successful breast-feeding is most likely when the parents have discussed the feeding of their infant prior to birth. Putting the infant to the breast soon after delivery and suckling on demand will usually establish the production of milk which is called lactation, but some women need help and encouragement to breast-feed. A peaceful atmosphere without distractions, and the assistance of a sympathetic and experienced person can be of immense benefit.

Some mothers prefer to feed their babies sitting up, others lying down. Do whatever is easiest and most comfortable for you. Also remember that each baby behaves differently at the breast. Some are always hungry, some excitable, while others seem sluggish or disinterested. But all babies have two important reflexes that you can use to help in feeding. The first is the 'rooting reflex' which is activated when baby smells the milk and senses the nipple near his mouth, he will move his head around trying to get hold of it. The 'sucking reflex' ensures that once he has the nipple or the teat of the bottle in his mouth he will automatically suck until the milk flows.

Most mothers, particularly after they have been nursing for a few weeks, have a distinct sensation of the milk being 'let down' at feeding time. This is partly due to milk filling the breast but it can also be stimulated by thinking about feeding or by hearing baby cry when he is hungry.

Many women feel miserable and inadequate a few days after birth and are apt to abandon breast-feeding because the milk supply seems insufficient or the let-down reflex is not yet functioning. Sometimes cracked nipples and engorged breasts cause pain and special treatment may be needed. It may be difficult for milk production to start if the infant is at first unable to suck because he is premature, sick or has some other problem. In these circumstances, the mother should try to express milk to stimulate and maintain a supply which can be given later to baby.

BREAST-FEEDING AT HOME

Nursing on demand is usually the most successful method of feeding as there is always considerable variation in the

All babies have two important reflexes that help in feeding
▼▼▼

quantity of milk taken and the frequency of feeds. Some infants at first take as many as twelve feeds in twenty-four hours, but most eventually accept a regular schedule with four or five feeds daily. Only rarely do breast-fed infants overfeed. Sometimes a rapid flow of milk may frighten an infant who will then scream and reject the breast. Slowing down the flow by hand and lying back so that the milk has to flow uphill may help, but expert advice may be needed. Poor initial flow, slow let-down reflex and nipples which are difficult for the infant to grasp may produce an angry, frustrated infant and an anxious, upset mother. Both of these will cause the milk supply to diminish rapidly. Sometimes a small additional bottle-feed may be needed for a short time to pacify the infant until the mother's confidence returns and the milk supply increases.

Breast-fed infants may be given extra fluids such as boiled water or diluted fruit juice. Extra fluids are usually unnecessary except in very hot weather or if an infant is ill with fever, vomiting or diarrhoea, but many mothers like to accustom their infants to an occasional bottle. Fluoride supplements to prevent tooth decay are generally not needed or recommended for breast-fed or bottle-fed babies where the water supply has fluoride added to it. If there is no fluoride added to the water, fluoride supplements should be used. But be careful not to give more than the recommended amount. This caution holds for vitamin supplements as well.

FORMULA-FEEDING

In an affluent society feeding with an appropriate formula is an easy alternative and bottle-fed infants thrive, develop normally and are just as well adjusted emotionally as breast-fed infants. It is important to hold baby close to you at feeding time to produce the same close body contact that occurs when a baby is breast fed.

Cow's milk must be diluted and suitably modified before being given to the young infant, and there are many excellent commercial preparations based on cow's milk which are modified to simulate human breast milk. Soya bean and goat's milk preparations are available for infants who are allergic to cow's milk or who cannot drink it for other reasons, though they are not needed for the vast majority of babies.

Infants may be bottle fed from birth, but preferably they should be given the first watery milk produced by the breast then gradually changed to formula-feeding. The breast milk produced in the first couple of days is known as colostrum. It contains substances which help to protect the baby against infection, and is very beneficial. Vitamins

Only rarely do breast-fed infants overfeed
▼▼▼

must be added if they have not been included in the milk preparation, and care must be taken to prepare the milk correctly. Bottle-fed infants, like breast-fed infants, should be demand fed. Overfeeding, obesity and faulty eating habits can occur more easily in artificially fed infants than in breast-fed infants.

FACTS AND FABLES ABOUT BREAST-FEEDING

Breast-feeding is valuable in a number of ways. Babies receive natural substances from the milk that help them resist various infections. Also, it saves hours of time each week because there are no bottles to sterilise, no formulas to mix, no refrigeration to worry about and no bottles to warm. But bottle-feeding does allow fathers to contribute to feeding and the work that it entails. Breast-fed babies rarely suffer from gastroenteritis. Perhaps the most important aspect of breast-feeding is the satisfaction that both mother and baby feels and the closeness and intimacy that develops between mother and baby. Some mothers are worried about breast-feeding because they feel it will spoil their figure. Certainly the breasts enlarge during pregnancy and in the early days of feeding, but a well-fitting nursing brassiere to support the breasts will prevent stretching of the skin and the breasts should return to their previous size and shape after feeding. Breast-feeding also stimulates the uterus to return to its normal size.

Some mothers feel that if they have small breasts, they will be less able to produce milk. There is no relationship between breast size and milk production. The size of the breasts is more related to fatty tissue than to milk-producing gland tissue.

There is an old wives' tale that breast-feeding 'takes a lot out of a mother'. Many young mothers feel fatigued, but this is rarely due to breast-feeding alone. A nursing mother must take sufficient extra kilojoules and nourishment to provide for her baby as well as for herself but, provided she is healthy and happy, her own appetite will take care of this.

The working mother presents another problem. However, if she wants to feed her baby, she can still do so except for the feedings that are required while she is at work. Creches and child-care centres may not be available in some workplaces but these help a working mother to continue to breast-feed.

Some mothers are concerned that what they eat or drink will affect baby. There is no evidence that tea, coffee or alcohol in moderation will harm baby. However, if you still smoke, this is a good time for you and your partner to stop forever. The closeness of a baby and his parents means that if either

Babies receive natural substances from breast milk that help them resist various infections
▼▼▼

parent smokes, baby will inhale quite a lot of smoke passively. There is good evidence that babies who are not exposed to cigarette smoke have fewer episodes of chest infection and asthma. Occasionally, a mother may find that some particular food does seem to upset baby. If this happens several times in succession, it's wise to cut down or stop eating this particular food until baby is weaned. Some medicines do get into milk, although not usually in significant quantities, but it's wise not to take any medicines while feeding baby unless you have discussed their use with your doctor. When a nursing mother becomes nervous or upset, it can affect the milk supply and it often seems to upset baby too.

The mother who takes this opportunity to build up a contented and secure relationship with her baby from the beginning starts with a great advantage. However, this may sometimes be impossible because of financial pressures, illness and other individual considerations. Clearly, there is no reason why a normal and healthy relationship between mother and baby should not develop when a baby is bottle fed.

FEEDING SCHEDULES

The question of demand feeding or adhering to a strict feeding schedule remains a matter of controversy, though today most paediatricians recommend demand feeding. In practice, it really makes very little difference. The baby fed by the clock and the demand fed baby will both settle down to a routine of approximate four-hourly feedtimes within a few weeks.

If your baby is small or particularly hungry, he may need feeding at more frequent intervals initially, but you should endeavour to get him settled into a schedule of approximately four hours once he is gaining weight and thriving.

There is no need to let baby rule your life entirely. If it's inconvenient to feed baby exactly four hours after the previous feeding, don't do it.

The amount of time taken for each feeding is also variable and depends very much upon the rate at which the milk flows and the avidity with which baby feeds. On average, about ten minutes to each breast seems to be right for most babies, but there is considerable individual variation. The usual practice is to let baby feed from both breasts at each feeding, starting with the left breast for one feed and the right for the next, and so on.

Most new mothers are worried about baby getting enough to drink. If baby appears content at the end of a feed, sleeps between feeds and is gaining weight at the normal rate, you can be sure that he is getting an adequate milk supply. If in

Most paediatricians recommend demand feeding
▼▼▼

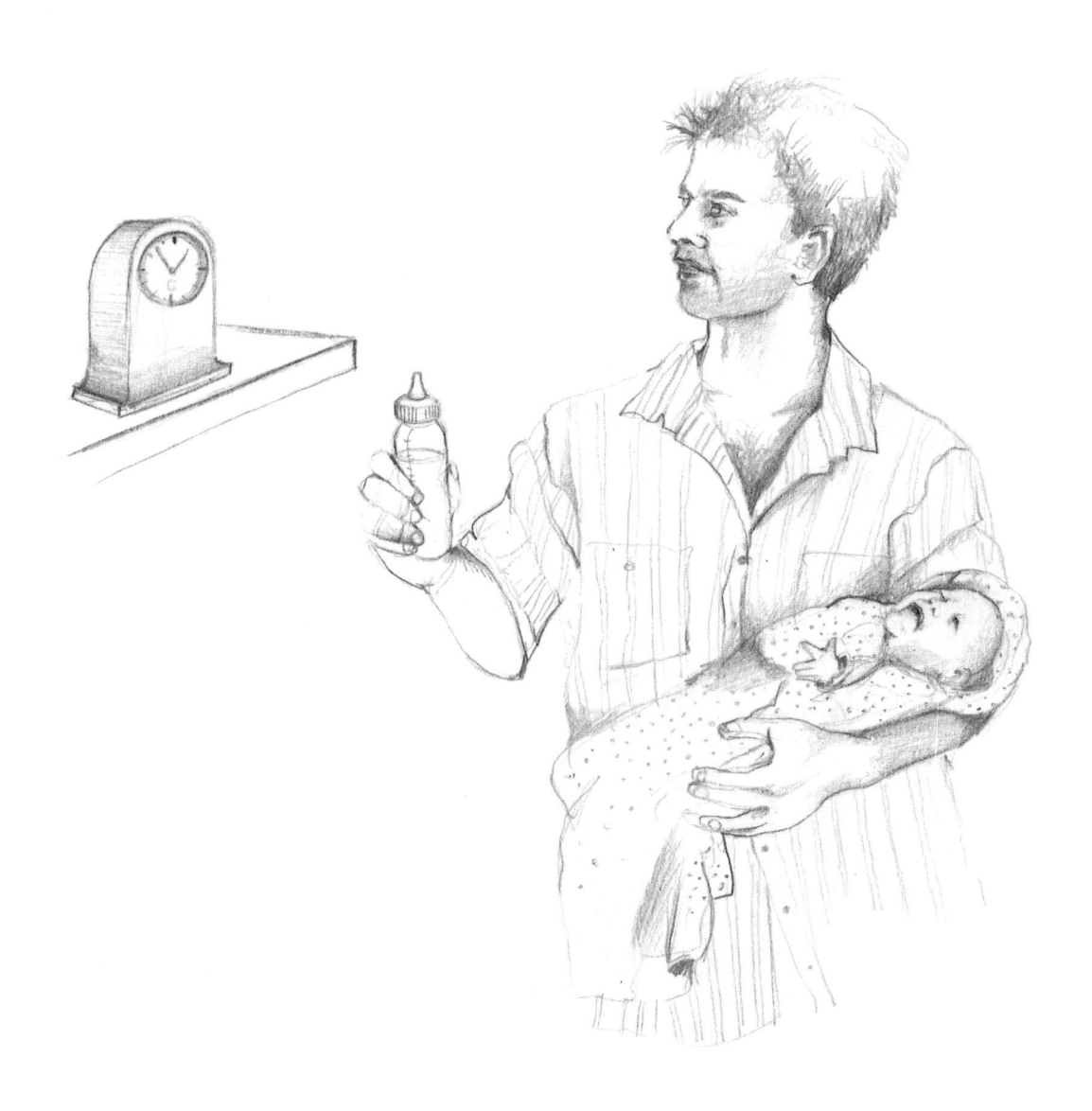

doubt, check with your clinic nurse and arrange to test weigh baby before and after feedings.

As baby gets a little older — around three months — you will find that you can eliminate the late-night feed. This will be a great relief to both parents. Some babies will naturally start to sleep through the night. If your baby does not, it is a good plan not to wake him after the six o'clock feeding in the evening and to let him sleep as late as possible. Feed him again at eleven or twelve o'clock and then see if he will sleep through until six in the morning.

Some feeding difficulties

Feeding difficulties may occur either in breast-fed or in formula-fed infants. If an infant screams a lot, especially at night, wind (or flatulence) in the stomach or the bowels, causing colic, is usually to blame. Changing the feeding will not help. Windy babies are usually active, complaining infants who need a lot of attention, and who don't like being hungry or tired, having wet nappies, having gas in the stomach or bowel, or being alone. They continue to thrive, but upset their parents and the whole family; they seem to need more body contact, cuddling and movement than a more placid infant. Professional advice may be needed, particularly if mother begins to feel tense, depressed and inadequate. Such infants seem to have extraordinary stamina, and can easily exhaust the whole family.

Some other infants vomit small amounts frequently, but still thrive. Propping the baby upright after feeds, the use of an agent to thicken the milk, or sometimes medicines help. If baby is thriving there is not much to worry about.

Cracked or inflamed nipples may make breast-feeding painful and unpleasant. Your obstetrician or family doctor or midwife will advise you about the care of the nipples during the last month of pregnancy. If your nipples crack and if feeding becomes painful, consult your doctor without delay.

Weaning

When the mother is producing only a small amount of milk there's usually not much trouble with weaning. If there's still a lot of milk, limiting fluid intake will usually help and baby can be allowed to feed on the breast for a brief period to reduce the pressure without stimulating the breast excessively. By decreasing the time that baby feeds and increasing the period between feeds, you'll find that the milk dries up quite quickly. At this stage, of course, baby will be taking most of his feedings from other sources. If sudden weaning is necessary, for instance if the mother or baby suddenly becomes ill, then special medical advice may be needed, but illness or anxiety about the baby will normally dry up the flow of breast milk.

Starting solids

Generally, it is better to delay solids until a baby is around five or six months old. From this age, most family foods are suitable to give baby. Here are a few points to keep in mind.

- It can be tempting to have baby reach milestones earlier than other babies, and to start on solids earlier than is necessary.

If baby is thriving there is not too much to worry about ▼▼▼

- Before six months of age, check carefully that what you may think is hunger in baby is not due to some other need, such as the desire for more playing or cuddling, or an infection starting.
- For the first year of life, your baby is dependent on milk for his basic food needs.
- For this reason it's a good idea to give him his milk before the solids until he's about nine months old. If you are breast feeding, this will also help keep up your milk supply. After this age you can offer him new foods at the beginning of his meal when he's hungry and, as a result, most likely to be willing to try something different.
- Within reason, keep to those foods which the family eats.
- There is really no need to add any sugar or salt to any of baby's foods.
- For the first spoon feed it is a good idea to hold baby in your arms, place a tiny amount of watery food on a spoon, then put this on the back of his tongue where it will have less chance of being spat back. Your baby will probably shudder at first!
- If he continually baulks at the spoon, provide him with finger foods instead.
- It is often best to wait a few days after offering a new food before starting another one; it's easier to detect food problems if there is a gap between the introduction of new foods.
- Don't start feeding problems by pushing or coaxing. Give him only what he wants, not what you think he should have.
- Beware of sweetening a food as a coax to 'get it down'. Extra sugar should be avoided.

FOOD SUGGESTIONS

SOME FIRST FOODS BABIES LIKE

Breakfast
- A good start is soft fruit, such as a banana, mashed with milk or water, then later just peeled and held in his hand. A rice based infant cereal is a good next step.
- He can hold and suck a rusk or a crust of bread, but it's wise never to leave him alone with any finger foods in case he chokes.
- Start using a cup with plain water or diluted but unsweetened fruit juice.

Lunch
- Try finely minced meat moistened with warm water, then later a piece of meat to suck, or a good sized chicken bone with a few pieces of meat attached — avoid bones that he might swallow.
- Egg yolk, soft boiled as a spoon feed, or hard boiled in a tiny sandwich can be tried, then soft fruit.

Offer him vegetables seperately, so that he learns about different tastes and textures
▼▼▼

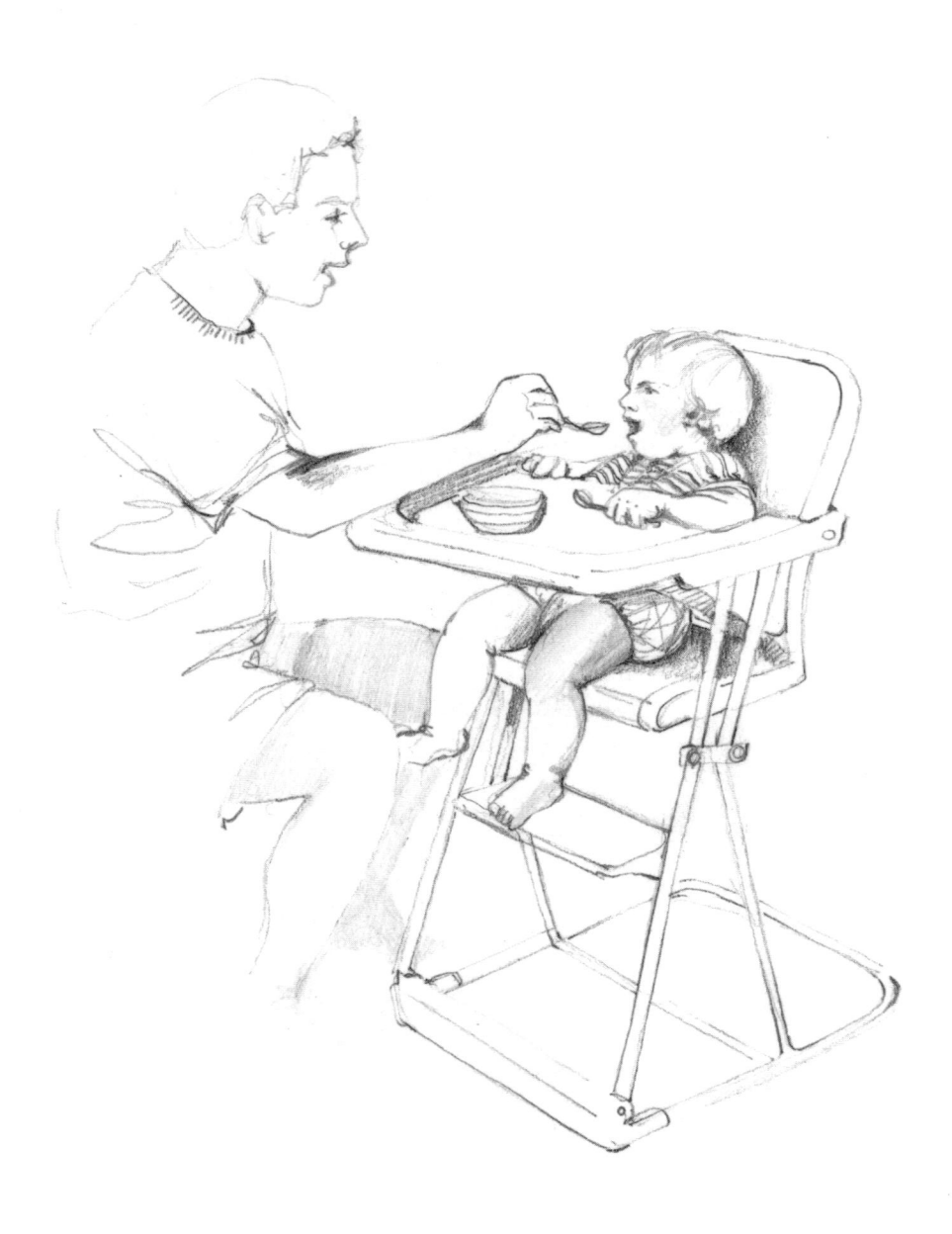

Tea
- Cook meat and vegetables without the addition of salt or sugar. Add these at the end of cooking for yourselves if necessary, but only after taking out a small serve for your baby.
- Offer him vegetables separately, not mashed together, so that he learns about different tastes and textures.
- Again, give him where possible unsweetened soft fruits and a plain dessert such as custard or yoghurt.
- It's a good idea to offer

something to chew on, as for lunch, then a cup of water or diluted fruit juice.

Meals for toddlers

Children, like adults, vary in their appetite and eat more on one day or at one meal than another. Don't make a toddler eat the same amount at each meal. Here is a selection of food suitable for toddlers.

Breakfast
- Cereal — porridge or ready-to-eat cereal, but no nuts or toasted cereal that could be inhaled. For that reason it's better not to use pre-mixed muesli.
- For variety, add fresh, stewed or dried fruit with cereal.
- Egg, mince, sausage, cheese or baked beans on toast.
- Toast and butter or margarine.
- Smooth peanut butter or a spread based on yeast or vegetable extract, such as Vegemite.
- Fruit juice or milk.

Morning tea
- Small sandwich (cheese, tomato, egg, and so on).
- Milk or juice.

Lunch
- Salad vegetables cut up, with meat, egg, cheese or a sandwich with any filling you fancy. Soup is a good alternative in cold weather, but be careful that it's not hot, only warm.
- Milk or juice.
- Bread and butter or margarine.
- Fresh fruit.

Afternoon tea
- Fresh or dried fruit.
- Juice or milk.

Tea
- Fish, meat, chicken, egg.
- Potato, rice or pasta.
- Vegetables (raw or cooked).
- Fruit (fresh or stewed).
- A dessert, such as custard or yoghurt.

Meals for kindergarten and school children

Once your child starts school, teachers and other children will influence his eating habits. What he sees on television will also influence him. Talk to him about things he would like to have for lunch rather than packing only what you think he should have. Send to school fresh fruit and packets of dried fruit for snacks.

Send to school fresh fruit and packets of dried fruit for snacks

▼▼▼

The new arrival 37

Fat Children and Thin Children

If both parents are fat it is unrealistic to expect the children to be slim
▼▼▼

Many parents worry that their child is too fat or too thin. There is a wide range of normality for weight and height. So long as your child falls within the normal range, you have no cause for concern. In any case, the common causes, such as heredity, temperament and appetite are outside your control. Your mother or mother-in-law may reassure you by saying that you or your partner were just like that as a small baby. Some children are always on the move and they burn up a lot of energy; others are placid, take little exercise and have more kilojoules left over to store as fat. The most important factor of all is appetite. Some children seem to be voracious eaters from birth and continue to have a big appetite. Other children show little interest in food and never want to eat a great deal.

If your child remains persistently undernourished and does not show a normal regular weight gain, or if there is a sudden loss of weight, you should consult your doctor. If the cause for this is not clear, consultation with a paediatrician is usually advisable.

Obesity can be a problem since it tends to continue into later life. It's difficult for fat children to enjoy exercise and games, so they tend to sit around instead of burning up energy. Also, fat children are likely to be the butt of jokes from other children and they turn to food for comfort. Many children tend to be naturally plump from about seven or eight through to puberty. At that stage, the greatest stimulus to weight reduction is the wish to be like others, especially like favourite media personalities, and the wish to be attractive to others.

If both parents are fat it is unrealistic to expect the children to be slim. Family eating habits are important and often difficult to alter.

If you think your baby is looking overweight, check on the following points in his diet and management.

1. Are you giving him extra cereals at teatime because he doesn't sleep through the night?
2. Is he having sweetened drinks — rosehip syrup, cordials, sweetened tinned fruit, sweet desserts, sugar on his cereal (even a tiny amount)?
3. Does he have honey or jam on his toast or bread?
4. Are you, or your child's grandparents or the baby-sitter, giving him chocolate or sweets, potato chips as a reward or to 'keep him quiet'?

FAT CHILDREN — WHAT CAN WE DO?

Treating obesity is always more difficult than preventing it. It is rarely necessary, or indeed possible, to put a child on a diet for weight reduction. It is sensible to substitute fresh fruit for puddings if your children tend to be on the plump side, and to substitute fruit or dried fruit for cakes, biscuits and bread as snacks. Encourage your child to participate in normal vigorous exercise. Swimming can often be a satisfactory substitute for the child who is disinclined to be involved in team sports.

The best idea is to always have available a large range of fresh fruits and dried fruits. Try to have a seasonal variety and buy less of the foods which will fatten the family. Have plenty of unsweetened fruit juice, chilled water, low-energy soft drinks and skim milk yoghurts in the refrigerator. Having unsuitable foods in the home will only cause unnecessary temptation. It's easier if everyone changes to a healthier diet.

WEIGHT REDUCING HINTS FOR MEALTIMES

Breakfast
- If your child is drinking cow's milk, modify it by substituting half of it with skim milk or a low fat milk, but don't exceed 600 ml of mixture daily.
- Allow a couple of weeks to cut out gradually all forms of sugar, and try to encourage a 'savoury tooth'.
- Use a little peanut butter on toast instead of honey or jam.
- Use only unsweetened fruit juices diluted by 50 per cent with water.

Morning tea
- Choose fruit that takes time to eat, such as pieces of apple.

Lunch
- Offer him a salad or a vegetable soup but be sure to include some protein like meat or chicken to satisfy his hunger. Don't buy fatty meats.

Afternoon tea
- Unsweetened fruit juice should be enough, or a small piece of fresh fruit.

Tea
- Choose lean cuts of meat and grill or roast it on a rack so that fat drips out of the meat. Don't use this for gravy.
- Don't add butter or margarine to his vegetables, which should be steamed or boiled.
- Offer unsweetened canned or stewed fruit, and unsweetened dessert, such as a natural yoghurt. If the fruit is sour, add a spice like cinnamon to the fruit while cooking.

Beware of nagging your overweight child
▼▼▼

SOME GENERAL HINTS

- Above all, beware of nagging your overweight child and of putting an undue emphasis on food. Avoid battles and try not to appear concerned. Beware of discussing his weight problem with others in front of him.
- Make time to play with him more, and offer him a variety of toys and games to interest him and preferably keep him active.
- Encourage him to drink plain water by setting an example yourself.
- Together with watching the quality and quantity of his food intake, try increasing his physical activity. Suggest short walks after tea, have him join in family ball games, encourage walks and picnic lunches at the weekends, go swimming, and so on.

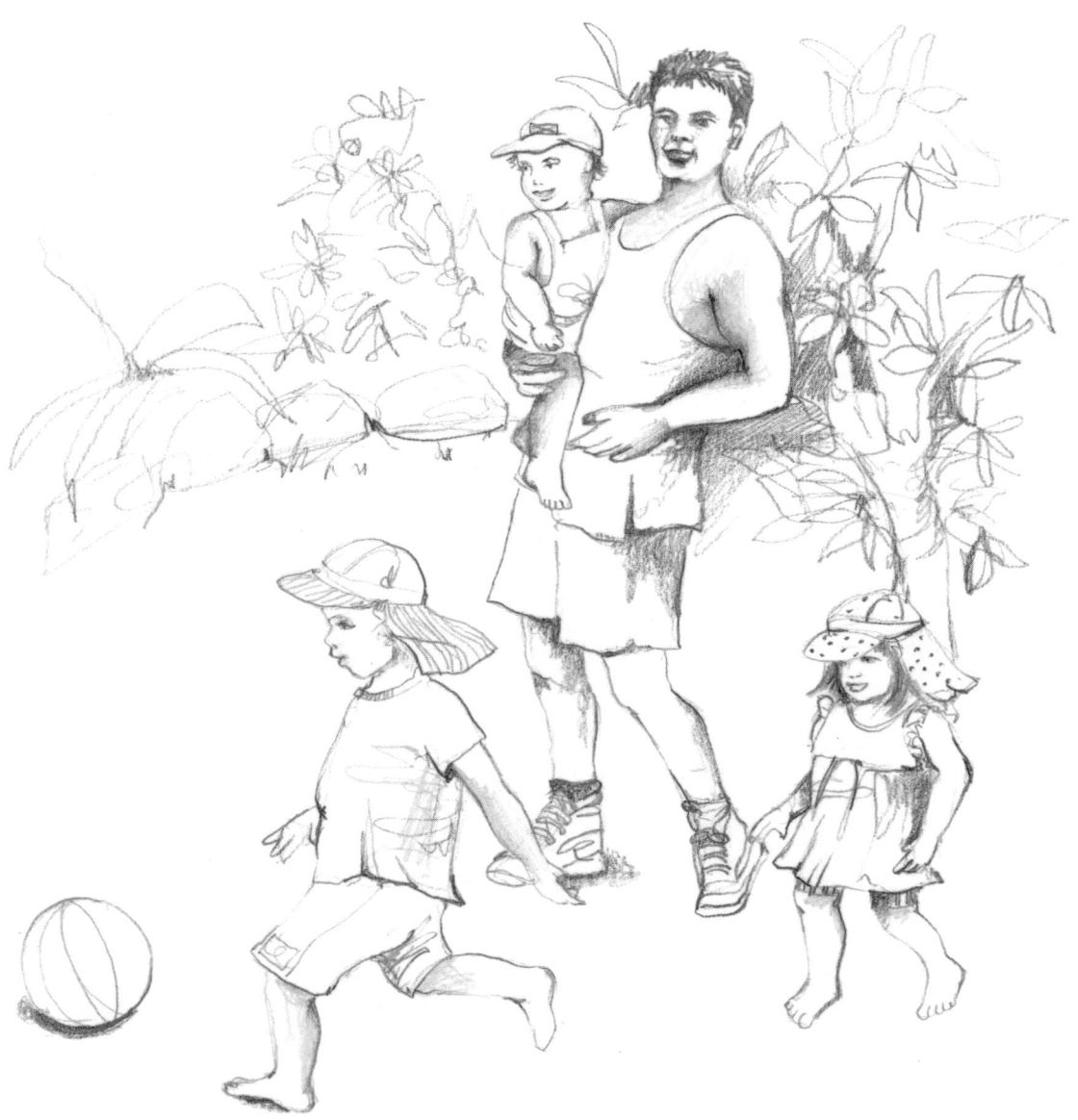

MEALTIME BATTLES

When a child refuses food many parents feel offended and react angrily because they're worried that their child is not eating enough — with the result the child continues to refuse and 'wins' the battle. It's always best to remain relaxed in these circumstances if your child is obviously well and growing normally. Nagging or bribing him will make him and you tense. Once a reasonable time has elapsed for the meal, it is best to put away all food; don't present the same dish at the next meal as a punishment!

Here are a few commonsense checkpoints if you and your child are continually clashing at mealtimes.

1. Children are very sensitive to atmosphere — mealtimes should be happy and relaxed.
2. Are your serves too big? Tiny servings with the option of seconds are better than one large serve.
3. Variety and colour are important, a different coloured plate or setting on occasions relieves monotony — try to have a meal outside or as a picnic on a rug.
4. Do you include favourite dishes and finger foods wherever possible?
5. Do you serve meals at fairly regular times? A tired child can quickly lose his appetite.
6. Indiscriminate eating between meals will obviously lessen the appetite for food at mealtimes, especially the eating or drinking of sugar foods or soft drinks.
7. Are your chairs and tables the right size, and comfortable for a child to sit on?
8. Keeping safety in mind, it's a good idea to let your child help with the meal preparation and cooking — fetching ingredients, doing simple measuring, stirring, rolling out pastry, and so on.
9. Have you tried inviting your child's special friend over to meals? It often works wonders!
10. Do you carry arguments over into mealtimes? It's always best to make the effort to make up with an unhappy child before a meal; eating then becomes a pleasure for you both.

Some children use mealtime battles as a means of asserting their developing independence.

It is important to understand this and not to allow mealtimes to become a trial of strength between you and your child. If he refuses his dinner after a reasonable time and a sympathetic approach, then desist, without any show of emotion, and wait for the next meal. Children never starve themselves to death.

It's a good idea to let your child help with meal preparation and cooking ▼▼▼

CHAPTER 4

MILESTONES

It is exciting to watch your child grow and develop. So much is happening. The most obvious early milestones are those related to physical development — gaining weight, reaching towards things, trying to roll over. However, you will soon see exciting changes in mental development too — the way your baby starts to remember things and people and how she relates to the world around her.

What you hear or read about child development is the average. There is considerable variation in the rate at which normal babies reach their milestones. Your baby may reach some milestones faster than average and may be slower than average in some other areas. This is usually unrelated to the baby's level of intelligence and is just part of the normal variation. However, children do tend to reach their main milestones such as sitting, standing and talking in the same definite order. Also, development does not progress at the same steady, regular rate. There may be times when the baby appears to be making little progress, then this is usually followed by a spurt in development. This applies just as much to mental development and social behaviour as to the physical milestones.

Development progresses from top to toe starting with eye movements, then head control and then progressively co-ordinating neck, arms and hands, trunk, then legs. At first, these movements look fairly clumsy but they gradually become more co-ordinated and precise.

HEIGHT AND WEIGHT

Most babies have doubled their birth weight by five or six months of age and will have trebled it by their first birthday. Weight gain slows down a little after this, with approximately 2.5 kg being gained in the second and also in the third year. About 2 kg are gained each year until puberty when a further growth spurt occurs. However, weight is not gained at the same steady rate throughout the year. Just as other aspects of development come in spurts, there may be times when your baby seems to have gained little weight over a one or two week period and other times when the weight gain may be quite impressive. The pattern of weight gain over a longer period is more important than changes occurring over a few days.

Length also increases most in the first six months so that by the first birthday your baby will be one and a half times her birth length. A child's ultimate height and weight are determined by a number of factors. Some are genetic, such as parent size, while others are environmental, such as food intake and general health. Future adult height and weight cannot be accurately predicted in the first few years of life. Plump babies do not necessarily result in fat adults. Babies are naturally plump, with this chubbiness reaching its maximum around the age of nine months. In the second and third years, when the infant is walking, running and generally more active, a leaner build will develop.

Seeing and Hearing

Babies can see right from the time of birth. They have a particular liking for faces and quickly respond to faces looking closely at them. By six to eight weeks babies will smile back to a smiling face and will also be smiling in response to any pleasurable stimulation. By three months many babies will be regularly distinguishing the face of mother and father from others and by six months may show some anxiety when they see a strange face that they do not recognise.

A baby's hearing is well developed for some months before birth. Right from birth baby will respond to the sound of a human voice, particularly a higher pitched female voice. By six months baby will be able to consistently localise a sound and will show delight when familiar, pleasurable sounds are heard.

Speaking

It's important to talk to your baby right from the very beginning. Even though it will be some time before your baby talks back, this early and regular experience of language is the basis for the baby's language development. Within a few weeks your baby will respond to your gentle language by murmuring, gurgling and squealing. By five or six months a tuneful, babbling language will have developed which, although quite incomprehensible, will have the rhythm of speech and will give you and the baby lots of pleasure as you talk to each other.

Although babies begin to understand the meaning of a lot of words towards the end of the first year, they may only be able to say one or two single words with meaning by the first birthday. Their ability increases rapidly after about eighteen months so that by the second birthday there may be a vocabulary of over one hundred words with some words starting to be joined together. By the age of four there will be more complicated sentences and most of the speech should be reasonably clear.

Babies are naturally plump, with this chubbiness reaching its maximum around the age of nine months
▼▼▼

BILINGUAL FAMILIES

When mother and father each speak a different language or dialect, or if their native language is not English, the children have a wonderful opportunity to become bilingual. Some parents are worried that speaking to their children in two different languages will confuse them and may produce emotional disturbances or cause them to stammer. This is not so. Around two years of age, such children will begin to recognise there are two different words for various objects and they can then begin to receive an explanation of the reason for this. As they progress, they will respond automatically in the language in which they are addressed. Sometimes the acquisition of language may be slightly delayed but this is a small price for the later advantages of being able to speak two languages.

SOCIAL AND EMOTIONAL DEVELOPMENT

Social behaviour starts to develop within a few weeks of birth. The baby gurgles and coos in response to other people and by three months will be starting to laugh and squeal, to identify the sounds and characteristics of her parents and to show pleasure when with them. By six months, having learnt to recognise her parents, she may cry or resist when picked up by a stranger. As she becomes more aware of the existence of others this fear of strangers is lost. By twelve months she obviously enjoys being with people and tries to join in their conversations. She responds to praise and likes to show off newly learnt skills such as trying to take off socks or clapping hands. By eighteen months she will be trying to help in household tasks by imitating what she sees her parents doing. She is very responsive to love and cuddling.

During the second year strong likes and dislikes for various foods may appear. This is a normal stage of development which need not develop into mealtime battles if you can be flexible and substitute different foods until the fad passes. By eighteen months, even though she can indicate needs such as thirst and hunger, she cannot yet remember concepts clearly and cannot decide what is right and wrong. It's best to be positive with her and not expect her to make choices. Tell her it is dinner time — don't ask her if she is hungry. Tell her that you are taking her out in the stroller — don't confuse her by asking if she wants to go shopping with mummy or stay with daddy.

Young children are very responsive to love and cuddling
▼▼▼

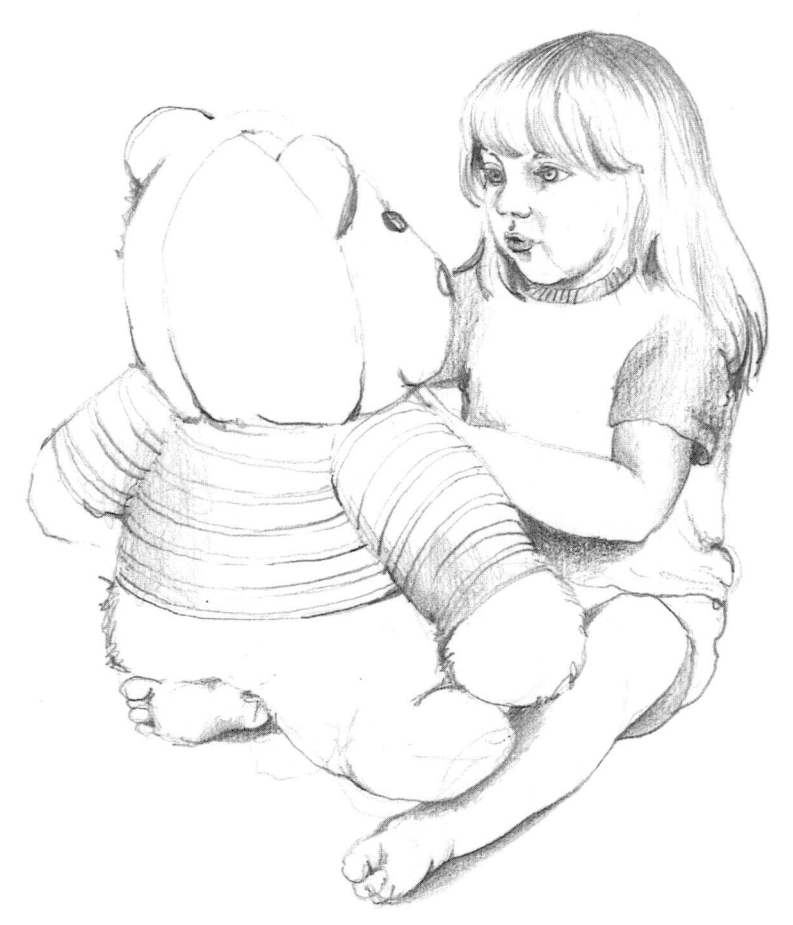

At this stage the child has no real concept of right and wrong or good and bad. She also has no clear concept of time. This means she won't understand if you tell her you'll be 'back later' as 'later' has no meaning for her. She may also become confused if given too many choices. She has a short concentration span, likes to play with one toy at a time but will quickly change from one toy to another. Promises and threats have no meaning at this age. It is useless to say to a two-year-old, 'If you don't touch the ornaments on the coffee table, you can have a biscuit'. It is much wiser and more effective not to have ornaments on the coffee table so that this and similar problems around the house don't arise. By the time she is two she will be starting to comprehend firm commands such as 'no' and 'don't touch', just as she will be responsive to praise and encouragement.

Between two and three, play becomes more complex. She will enjoy piling blocks on top of each other to make a tower and start to actively participate in games, as long as she is the centre of attention. At this age, many children start to treat a special

Milestones 45

Young children do not deliberately lie
▼▼▼

doll or teddy bear as a real person, wanting it present at meal and bath time and taking it to bed. For some children, a soft piece of cloth or a baby blanket becomes an inseparable companion. These special toys or comforters are very important to the child, especially in new and strange situations, such as sleeping in a strange bed or going to hospital. Their affection for these objects should be respected as they seem to be an important mechanism that many children of this age use to help cope with the world around them.

As your child's language develops, so does her power of imagination. You will notice that her play becomes very creative and imaginative and that she can have a marvellous time by turning a couple of old boxes into a house or a ship. Occasionally your child will tell you the most amazing stories where imagination and the real world seem to be mixed up, although you will usually find there is an element of truth to the story. It's helpful to realise that children of this age do not deliberately lie and certainly should not be punished for these stories, although you should be starting to teach them from an early age, by personal example as well as by words, the importance of being truthful.

By around three years of age children start to need the company of other children more and more. This is a good age to introduce them to a neighbourhood playgroup or start them attending a kindergarten. As well as getting children used to their own age group, these experiences help them to develop social skills, to become less dependent on the same adult for everything and to start getting used to living in a world where not everything exists just for their own benefit.

Between two and three years children often become frustrated when they can't get their own way or because they can't get their bodies to do the complicated activities they think they ought to be able to do. This often leads to temper tantrums or occasionally to breath holding. Tantrums are best ignored, although this is not always easy. If you give the child what she wants because she's having a tantrum, the child quickly learns that a tantrum can be a very effective way of getting her own way. Dealing with tantrums by ignoring them, preferably by leaving the room so that the child no longer has an audience, soon teaches the child that there's nothing to be gained by having a tantrum. A breath holding episode can be quite frightening for parents. The child holds her breath so effectively that her lips and tongue turn deep blue. In some cases the child may go limp and faint. The good news is that although breath holding looks frightening to parents it is quite harmless to the child.

Deal with tantrums by ignoring them
▼▼▼

Breath holding is best dealt with in the same way as tantrums.

BLADDER AND BOWEL CONTROL

By about eighteen months to two years your child should be ready to start toilet training. It is not until this age that infants have matured enough to be aware of the sensation of bladder or bowel fullness and to communicate this to their parents. You may meet other parents who claim to have toilet trained their baby under one year. What they have really done is to take advantage of their baby's normal reflexes. Babies tend to pass a bowel motion automatically after a feed, and if placed on the pot at this time, or often enough in between, the impression will be given that they are toilet trained even though they are not able to indicate their needs or have any real control over their bowels or bladder.

A good indication of when to start toilet training is when your baby makes some indication by a sound, word or action, such as pulling at the nappy, that the nappy is about to, or has just become dirty. This is the time to start using a pot or training chair. These are better than a special seat on the toilet as a motion can be passed more easily when the feet are firmly on the floor and some babies are frightened of the height of a toilet seat. It may be some time from when toilet training starts until control is achieved. If the child resists your attempts to get him to use the pot, don't use force. Toilet training should not, and will not, become a battle of wills if the child is introduced to the pot gradually and praised when it is used. It's best not to start toilet training at times of stress, such as when the child is ill or when a new baby arrives in the home.

From around three years of age most children should have bladder and bowel control during the day although accidents may still occur, especially when they are absorbed in play or occasionally when there are times of stress. Bed-wetting often continues for another year or so, with close to 20 per cent of five-year-olds still wetting at night.

TEETH

There are two sets of teeth, the temporary 'milk' teeth and the permanent teeth, the first of these being the six-year-old molars. Rarely a tooth may be present at birth but the usual time for them to start to appear is at around six months, starting with the two lower teeth, called the lower central incisors. During the next six months a total of eight incisors appear, followed by the first double teeth (molars) between

It may be some time from when toilet training starts until control is achieved
▼▼▼

Teething has no relationship to the baby's other milestones or to the baby's level of intelligence ▼▼▼

twelve and eighteen months. Then come the eye teeth, then the second molars, sometimes called the two-year-old molars. Teething is a milestone which has no relationship at all to the baby's other milestones or to the baby's level of intelligence. In one infant the first tooth may proudly appear at three months, in another it may not appear until the first birthday, yet both may be perfectly healthy, normal babies.

The care of your baby's teeth should start well before the baby is born. This is because the tooth buds form quite early in pregnancy and is one of the reasons expectant mothers should have plenty of milk, fresh fruit and vegetables to provide the nutrients needed for good teeth development. The time when that first tiny tooth appears is the time to start tooth cleaning using a soft toothbrush. From about two years of age children should be encouraged to start cleaning their own teeth, something which can easily be done if you make a game of it and get the child to imitate you as you clean your teeth. However, children don't develop the co-ordination to clean their teeth properly until five or six, so you will need to check them for the child by cleaning them again. Use a fluoride toothpaste even when there is fluoride in the water supply. A great deal has been written about fluoride over the years. The truth is that when the water supply has fluoride added no harm has resulted and children have had a marked reduction in dental problems. If flouride is added to the water supply, additional flouride tablets should not be given.

It's a good idea to take your child to the dentist for a check-up at three or four years of age and to start regular checks from this time. Looking after the milk teeth helps the permanent teeth come through in their correct position. You can also reduce dental decay by not giving your child many sweet, sticky foods (instead give fruit, cheese, celery sticks and carrot sticks as snacks) and by cleaning the teeth promptly after eating sugary foods.

Teething is something that all parents seem to have been warned about and which gets unnecessarily blamed for a variety of problems. However, teething can cause some discomfort. The appearance of the tooth may be preceded by drooling, wanting to bite on rattles and toys and sometimes irritability. Sometimes the bowel actions may become a little loose. However teething never causes serious problems. If your child becomes really sick when teething, such as with a high fever, profuse diarrhoea or listlessness, see your doctor quickly as these sorts of symptoms may mean there is a more serious problem.

Because babies who are teething like to chew on things,

avoid giving them toys made of brittle plastic which could break in the baby's mouth. A rubber teething ring is much safer.

FEET

Parents often wonder about whether their child's feet are shaped normally and even when to start their baby off in shoes. Babies don't really need anything on their feet except for booties when it's cold. They don't need shoes until they are walking, although there is nothing wrong with letting them walk and run with bare feet some of the time. Shoes should be wide enough so that the toes are not crowded together.

All babies have relatively flat feet to start with. You will notice that the place where the arch would be is fat and chubby. The arch gradually becomes more defined as the child starts to stand and walk. Although many children in their earlier years look as if they may be developing pigeon toes or knock-knees, this is usually not the case. Almost all infants have some bowing of the legs which has usually corrected itself by two years. At about three years many children have some degree of knock-knee, often accompanied by the toes pointing inwards. This also corrects itself spontaneously, usually by five or six years, and only needs treatment in rare cases. Special shoes or shoes with build-ups are rarely required.

IMMUNISATION

Immunisation has saved countless lives. You may occasionally hear stories of the dangers of immunisation. Most of these stories have little factual basis. While it is true that no immunisation is 100 per cent effective or 100 per cent free of side-effects, modern immunisations are highly effective and very safe. There are some genuine, but rare, medical reasons for not immunising, but for parents, it is part of their parental responsibility to take their children to be immunised. Your doctor will tell you if there is any reason to avoid immunisation. The National Health and Medical Research Council puts the case for immunisation clearly and firmly: 'No children should be denied immunisation without serious thought about the consequences, both for the individual child and community'.

DIPHTHERIA, PERTUSSIS (WHOOPING COUGH) AND TETANUS

Immunisation against these three diseases is done with a single injection (triple antigen) given at

All babies have relatively flat feet to start with
▼▼▼

Milestones

Have your baby immunised at a time when she is well ▼▼▼

two, four, six and eighteen months with an extra booster against diphtheria and tetanus at five years. Have your baby immunised at a time when she is well although minor sniffles are not a reason to delay immunisation. Check with your doctor.

POLIOMYELITIS (POLIO)

This vaccine is given by mouth at two, four and six months (at the same time as triple antigen) with a booster at five years. It should not be given to children when they have diarrhoea as this impairs its efficiency.

MEASLES, MUMPS AND RUBELLA (GERMAN MEASLES)

As measles can be a serious disease, all children should be protected by measles immunisation. This is done at twelve months of age by a single injection which also gives protection against mumps and rubella. About one child in seven will develop a fever five to ten days after the immunisation and about one in twenty will have a mild rash. The protection this immunisation gives against mumps prevents the serious complications which can occur in some children who suffer from it. Rubella immunisation means that when your daughter grows up and starts to have children of her own, the risk of her unborn baby being infected with rubella, which can cause heart defects, deafness and blindness, is virtually eliminated.

HAEMOPHILUS INFLUENZA TYPE B (HIB)

Haemophilus influenza type B is a bacteria which can cause serious illnesses such as meningitis and a dangerous throat infection called epiglottitis. The immunisation, called HIBTiter, is given at two, four, six and eighteen months of age. Because Aboriginal children are more susceptible to HIB infection, they should be immunised at two, four and twelve months using a vaccine called PedvaxHIB.

HEPATITIS B

This immunisation, which protects against one of the more serious types of hepatitis, is not routinely given to all babies. Your doctor will advise you as to whether hepatitis immunisation is needed for your baby. It is given by three injections, the first soon after birth, the second at one month and the third at six months.

IMMUNISATION SCHEDULE

This chart gives the immunisation schedule recommended by the Australian National Health and Medical Research Council.

RECOMMENDED CHILDHOOD IMMUNISATION SCHEDULE

Age	Disease	Immunisation
2 months	• diphtheria, tetanus, pertussis • poliomyelitis • infections due to haemophilus influenza type B	• triple antigen 'DTP' • oral Sabine vaccine • *HIB vaccine
4 months	• diphtheria, tetanus, pertussis • poliomyelitis • infections due to haemophilus influenza type B	• triple antigen 'DTP' • oral Sabine vaccine • HIB vaccine
6 months	• diphtheria, tetanus, pertussis • poliomyelitis • infections due to haemophilus influenza type B	• triple antigen 'DTP' • oral Sabine vaccine • HIB vaccine
12 months	• measles, mumps, rubella	• measles–mumps–rubella 'MMR'
18 months	• diphtheria, tetanus, pertussis • infections due to haemophilus influenza type B	• triple antigen 'DTP' • HIB vaccine
5 years or prior to school entry	• diphtheria and tetanus • poliomyelitis	• combined diphtheria–tetanus 'CDT' • oral Sabine vaccine
10–16 years (females only)	• rubella (preferably in last year of primary school or first year of high school)	• rubella vaccine
15 years or prior to leaving school	• diphtheria and tetanus	• adult diphtheria and tetanus 'ADT'

*Aboriginal children should be immunised against HIB infection at two, four and twelve months.

Milestones

Travelling with Children

Travelling with small children needs considerable advance planning
▼▼▼

Long trips are now commonplace for business and for holidays. Very often the trip will mean visiting a foreign land where customs will be different, so it's worth devoting some time to the planning.

Travelling with small children particularly needs considerable advance planning. If a long journey by car is involved, plan to break it up into short stages, with an opportunity for the children to get out and run around to work off some of their extra energy. Plan for some suitable games to pass the time on the journey. Ensure that each child has her own safety seat or safety belt, suitable for her age and size. Young children should not to be carried in the front seat.

Feedings require careful planning. Take a supply of prepared baby foods, if appropriate, and make sure you have a portable cooler for food storage. Children tend to be creatures of habit and they will respond much better to their usual breakfast cereal than to something strange. Make sure you have plenty of their favourite cold drink with you in summer. When it is necessary to buy food en route, make sure it's fresh, and if in doubt, it's safer to bring fresh fruit and milk in sealed containers.

If one particular child is prone to car sickness and she is over eight years, she will usually travel better in the front seat, but like adults she must wear a seat belt.

With small infants, take a good supply of disposable nappies unless you know that you can purchase them en route. A large box of disposable tissues saves washing numerous handkerchiefs as well as being handy for a variety of emergencies. A supply of pre-moistened towelettes or a wet facecloth in a plastic bag is also useful. With a small baby, two or three large sheets of plastic sheeting will have a variety of uses, and don't forget that most important utensil — the potty. If your child has a special toy or a cuddly, it's important to take that with you, too.

If your trip is going to take more than one day it's wise to agree in advance that you will start looking for suitable accommodation by 4 p.m. rather than pressing on grimly with tired, irritable children. However, in school holidays, it is wise to book your accommodation in advance.

Many parents worry about the psychological effects on the children of long trips, particularly out of the country. Providing you move as a family unit you need have no particular concern. If you are travelling by air, all the major airlines make special provision for small children, but it's wise to let them know well in advance. If you have a small infant they may often give you a seat immediately behind one of the bulkheads where an airline bassinette can be hung.

With regard to feeding, school and daily activities, try to settle into a normal routine as soon as possible after arrival.

If you are travelling around with young children while you are away, particularly in the United Kingdom and Europe where the distances are relatively small, a caravan or campervan can have considerable advantages over trying to cope with hotels, strange foods and language difficulties with small children in tow.

When travelling in the tropics beware of buying food from open street stalls, even though locals seem to do it with immunity. Carry a knife and spoon with you to peel your own fresh fruit and to eat freshly prepared melons. If it's difficult to wash your hands beforehand, carry some pre-moistened tissues with you.

Some bandaids and some antiseptic paint or cream are useful for superficial cuts and abrasions. A little care in this regard may save later troubles.

Most airlines or governmental health agencies will give you advice about the health hazards of any foreign countries you are visiting. Ask them specifically about vaccinations against infectious diseases prevalent in the region where you may be travelling.

A supply of premoistened towelettes is useful
▼▼▼

CHAPTER 5

GROWING UP

EARLY RELATIONSHIPS BETWEEN MOTHER AND BABY

We know that early and continuing contact between mother and baby helps to establish a valuable bond that is important in a child's subsequent development. In many less industrialised societies, not only is baby enveloped and protected by the mother during development, but after birth babies tend to be slung close against their mothers for long periods as they go about their regular activities. Our 'developed' society sometimes puts barriers between mother and child, and it's only in recent years that we have realised how important it is to maintain the intimate relationship that has always existed in some other societies.

We know that early and continuing contact between mother and baby helps establish this bonding relationship. Skin contact is important while you are bathing and dressing your infant. Breast-feeding helps. This does not mean that the bottle-fed baby or the premature infant who is enclosed in an incubator for the first weeks of life cannot establish a successful relationship, but it does mean that mothers of such infants will need to take special care to compensate for the loss of this early, close and intimate relationship which normally lays the foundation for those special feelings of love and trust which exist between a mother and her child.

All of the following recommendations can be helpful in reinforcing that most important unit of modern society — the family. However, bear in mind that all these decisions are individual and personal. We suggest you discuss them and think about them and then make up your own minds — they are options not obligations.

- Fathers should be able to, and be encouraged to, attend the birth.
- Both mother and father should have their baby to hold and cuddle as soon as possible after it is born. Usually your baby will sleep in a bassinette next to you in the hospital.
- Breast-feeding should be strongly recommended but a mother should not be made to feel guilty if for any reason she cannot or does not wish to breast-feed her baby.

- Mothers should be encouraged to handle and fondle their babies right from birth and to look after them themselves as much as possible.

RELATING TO OTHERS

The young infant can relate to and progressively identify a limited number of other people. Firstly mother, then father, brothers and sisters. From the age of about six months, you will start to notice baby's growing sense of individuality and his progress towards the achievement of independence. Although parents are by far the most important, especially at first, growing up involves a gradual progression from total dependence to self-reliance. The important thing is that it should be gradual and progressive, making allowance for any setbacks that may occur, due to such situations as illness or unavoidable separation.

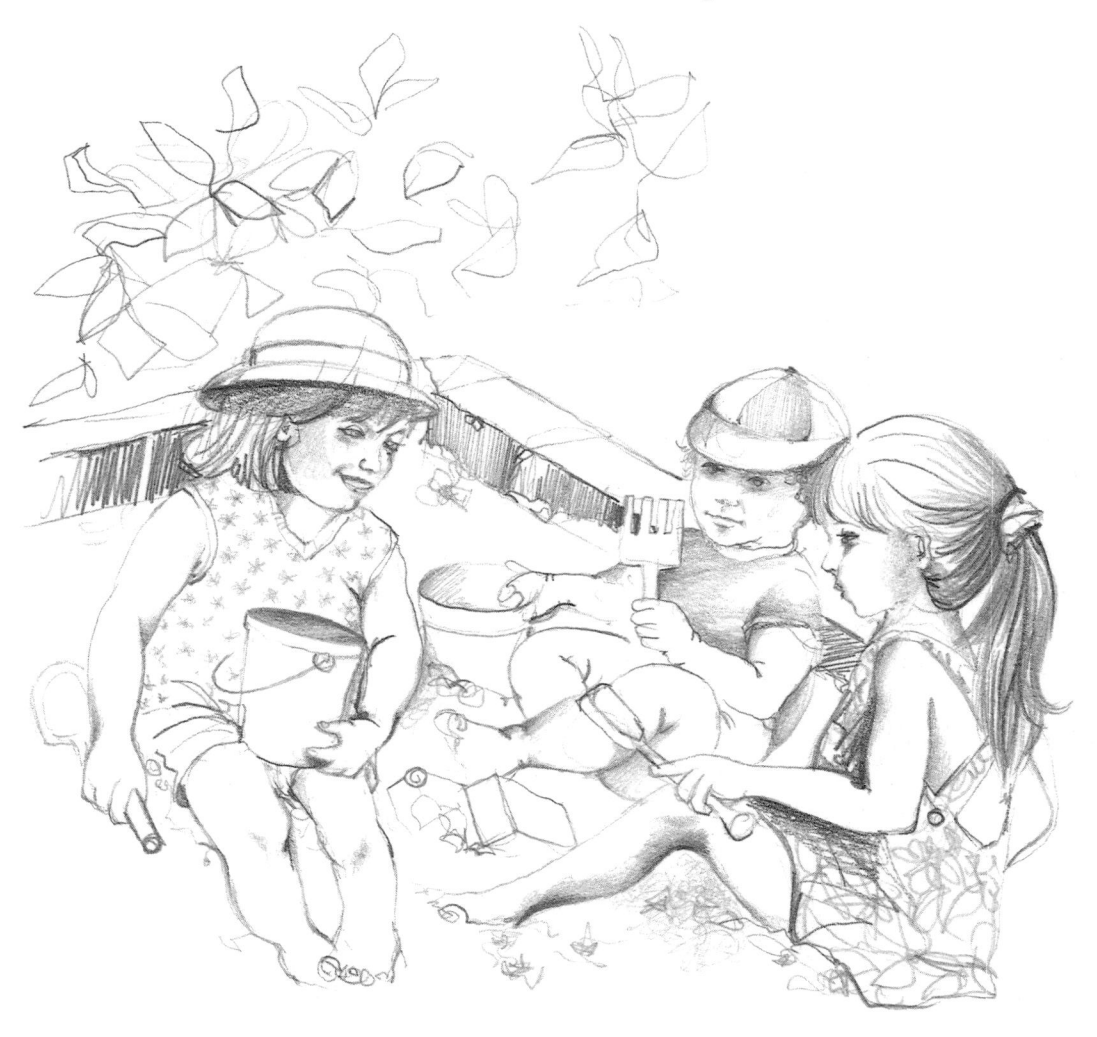

Growing up

SEPARATION

Adults and most older children can tolerate some separation quite readily. We can anticipate the future more or less effectively. We can accept explanation and reassurance, and most of us are able to come to terms with those losses that are inevitable. However, the young child has none of the adult's sophisticated ways of coping with separation.

One of the normal ways in which infants reveal this anxiety is in fear of strangers, usually evident around six to eight months of age. As your child develops the ability to recognise and identify individuals with whom he comes into frequent contact, such as neighbours and close relatives and friends, he tends to lose his fear of strangers. This usually occurs between twelve and eighteen months of age. Other ways in which your baby may show that he is afraid of being separated from his parents are in sleep disturbance, either in the form of refusal to go to bed or intermittently waking and crying during the night. His needs at this time are for reassuring support with as much secure contact with mother and father as possible.

It is worth stressing the importance of fathers. However, in most family situations, your child soon learns that he 'loses' his father from early in the morning until just before he goes to bed at night. He soon comes to identify the weekend as a special time when Dad is also available during the day. It's important that fathers recognise that fathering is just as important as mothering in the development of their child.

Just as your baby rapidly adjusts to the daily absence of a parent and the fact that the parent regularly reappears before bedtime, in the same way he learns to gradually adjust to temporary separation from his mother. The start along the important road to independence commences — both for him and for you — when you are able to leave him in the care of another responsible adult without distress on his part or yours. It's best if this is with somebody your baby already knows and trusts, such as a grandparent or one of your close friends.

DEATH IN THE FAMILY

It is difficult for an adult to understand exactly what death means to a child. By the age of three or four a child's imagination has developed to the stage where it's possible for him to envisage situations that he has not actually experienced. His picture of such situations will often be distorted and will initially tend to be drawn

As your child develops the ability to recognise close relatives and friends, he tends to lose his fear of strangers
▼▼▼

from picture books, fairy stories and his own familiar environment. The death of an older member of the extended family, particularly if it has been preceded by a period of illness, can be handled without too much difficulty. If the family has a religious background this will obviously be part of the explanation. If, however, death involves a parent or another close member of the family, the effect on a child can be devastating. It is impossible to generalise about such a situation apart from the obvious need to be intensely supportive and to seek appropriate professional help if necessary.

However, it's important to be honest with the child and not to make the mistake of trying to pretend nothing serious has happened. He should be allowed to express his grief, to attend the funeral if he wants to, and be given credit for having real emotions which he may want to pour out at this time.

It is always tempting to tell children to cheer up, but we must remember that there are times when children have a need to be sad, and they need help and understanding in coping with their grief. Handling grief is not a matter of forgetting and reminders of happy memories are important.

Remember that death is a natural part of life and children should not be prevented from sharing in the family mourning. It is, however, sensible to ask a child what he would like to do.

BABY-SITTERS

While the arrival of a new baby, particularly the first one, is a very important event for the family, mothers and fathers still need to set aside time for each other. Sometimes you will need a baby-sitter.

If you don't have someone you already know, it's best that you and your child have had an opportunity to meet the baby-sitter so that you feel confident that this is a person who gets on well with children, and can manage them capably, with kindness and understanding. This will also give your child a chance to get to know the new baby-sitter so that, should he wake up while you are out, he will not be faced with a stranger.

It is preferable for baby-sitting to be done in your home although this may not always be possible, rather than for the child to be left in strange surroundings. Before you go out, make sure that your baby-sitter knows where everything is that might be needed, and any special words that your child uses, such as when he wants to go to the toilet. Also, let your baby-sitter know what time you expect to be back and where you can be reached.

There are times when children have a need to be sad, and they need help and understanding in coping with their grief
▼▼▼

Growing up 57

Leaving your child in the care of a sensible and responsible person in this way from time to time not only allows you to lead a fuller and more satisfying life and to retain contact with friends, but it also plays a part in your child's development and helps him to become less dependent on you in a normal, healthy and progressive manner.

Common behaviour problems

Many of the common behaviour problems are merely reactions to the various anxieties and frustrations that children encounter while they are learning to master various new skills, or as they learn that the world wasn't created entirely for their benefit after all and that they cannot always have their every wish satisfied immediately. Others relate to infantile activities associated with pleasure or comfort, while others relate to their natural curiosity about their own bodies and their immediate environment.

Thumb sucking

Almost all babies suck their fingers or thumbs at some stage. In some children the habit persists for many years, particularly when they are tired or shy. Infants suck their thumb because it helps them to recapture the sense of comfort and security they originally experienced during suckling. This 'oral gratification' plays an important part in an infant's life, something you will notice when your baby is between six and twelve months of age, when everything is automatically popped into the mouth.

There have been all sorts of suggestions about the significance of thumb sucking — that it is more common in bottle-fed babies that are allowed only a limited time at the breast, that it is an indication of insecurity or maladjustment, and so on. The truth is that thumb sucking disturbs parents and well-meaning relatives a lot more than it does children. It's much better and less disturbing to let them stop the habit of their own accord. Many children will stop spontaneously by the age of about three. By then they are usually dissuaded by the fact that their friends don't do it and they don't like to be different. Above all, don't use any form of restraint, such as splints or mittens, because the frustration caused by these unnecessary measures is much more harmful than the habit itself. The same applies to punishing or forcefully removing the thumb from the mouth.

Many common behaviour problems are reactions to anxieties and frustrations that children encounter
▼▼▼

Dummies

There are no real objections to dummies as long as they are kept clean. However, if you are worried about your child sucking his thumb, by all means give him a dummy for a few months instead.

Many parents are worried that thumb sucking or the use of a dummy will distort the child's teeth. If they have any effect at all it's a very minor one and then only on the first teeth. By the time the permanent teeth come through, the habit has ceased and can have no possible effect on them.

Comforters

Just as some babies find comfort and security in thumb sucking, others develop a deep attachment to a particular object from which they obviously obtain considerable comfort. Sometimes, this is a soft toy such as a rag doll or teddy bear. More frequently, it's a piece of blanket or soft cloth which must be with them before they'll settle down to sleep. Occasionally, the attachment is so intense that they carry their comforter around with them. More frequently, however, they just want it next to them in bed at night. The length of this attachment varies. In some children it is only a few months, in others it persists for several years. As with thumb sucking, there is no reason to break a child's attachment to his comforter. Sooner or later he will discard it naturally. No harm can result from letting a child become dependent on his cuddly comforter, and in any case you can't prevent it from happening. Like thumb sucking, it might worry you but it provides your baby with a lot of comfort and security. Little children tend to associate the objects that give them satisfaction with the people they love and to whom they feel closest. The comforter, whether it's a cuddly piece of soft blanket or rag, or a special toy, provides the link between a parent who cannot always be there and the child's natural anxiety and uncertainty about the large, strange world around him.

Other comforting habits

Some babies, when they are tired, will rock rhythmically, nod or roll their heads from side to side or even bang their head repeatedly. These rhythmic movements seem to comfort them and help them go off to sleep. They are of no special significance and usually disappear after a few months.

Infantile colic

This is a term used for the fussy, distressed crying which usually occurs in the evening, and which occurs in some babies in the first three months of life. Occasionally,

As with thumb sucking, there is no reason to break a child's attachment to his comforter

▼▼▼

Growing up

it can persist for four to five months. Sometimes it is caused by air which is swallowed during feeding and which stretches the upper bowel. Burping a baby after feeding sometimes helps to get rid of this air. However other babies have colic without any apparent cause. It is not due to hunger and usually not caused by changing the amount or type of feeding.

Many infants who have colic seem to be tense and restless. They startle easily and are very active. They may do best on a quiet regime; a quiet room, not too much stimulation and being wrapped up firmly. Using a dummy sometimes helps. The cries of a baby with colic can be very distressing and frustrating for parents. Unfortunately, medicines seem to make very little difference. Some parents find that rocking the baby gently can be soothing, while others find that a drive in the car seems to be the most effective way to settle the baby.

In spite of their excessive activity and crying, these babies usually thrive. You can obtain some comfort from the knowledge that the condition progressively improves from around three months of age.

Sleep disturbances

The sleeping pattern of some infants can be very frustrating. Individual sleep patterns vary greatly, some children sleep a great deal and others wake frequently. Sometimes sleep problems can be made worse if the baby is immediately picked up and cuddled or even played with whenever he starts to rouse. Most babies rouse several times during the night but then go back to sleep. However, if they learn that people pick them up and do nice things for them every time they wake, this may become the beginning of a sleep problem.

It's wise to have a regular bedtime, not to stimulate or excite the baby just before bedtime and to try to establish a regular night-time routine. If your child wakes, or protests on being put down, wait two or three minutes to see if he settles by himself. If he doesn't, return, comfort him gently by touch or by voice and then leave the room. If the crying recommences, you can now wait three to four minutes before going in. You can repeat this process, gradually lengthening the time. Most infants learn to settle themselves down to sleep within a week using this technique which is far preferable to deciding one night to let your baby 'cry it out'.

Wakefulness in toddlers

This can occur for a variety of reasons. One of these is fear of separation, coupled with the toddler's fertile imagination,

It's wise to have a regular bedtime and to establish a regular night-time routine
▼▼▼

which may lead to reluctance to be left alone in the dark. The best treatment for separation anxiety is prevention. Allow your child to gradually develop some independence by leaving him for short periods with someone he knows and trusts, secure in the knowledge that you will always return. Anxiety about the dark can often be overcome by leaving a radio softly playing near the child's bed, or by using a small night-light.

There are a number of other minor bedtime problems in this age group. One is 'I want a drink of water', another 'I want to do wee wee'. If your child is really smart he will alternate the two. A third difficulty is the two to three year old who has learnt to climb out of his cot as soon as he is put to bed and reappears in the lounge room for a chat and a cuddle.

Patience, firmness and consistency are the answer for these problems. Getting up should not be allowed to pay off as an adventure or as a pleasurable experience. A quick cuddle, by all means, if you feel that reassurance is needed, but then a firm understanding that it's back to bed and off to sleep. If the condition persists, a discussion with your doctor may be advisable and sometimes mild sedation for a few nights may induce the sleep habit. Don't be tempted to use any form of restriction. Never fasten a child in bed with a harness or use any form of net or restriction over the cot and don't lock the bedroom door.

Temper tantrums

Anger is a normal response to frustration at any age. Most toddlers have not yet learnt to contain their anger and have not developed any sophisticated ways of expressing it. Also, some children become more easily frustrated than others and learn that tantrums are a way of getting what they want. Some children take the simplest direct approach. They lie on the ground and yell, beating it with fists and feet. In the majority of children these tantrums quickly cease with increasing maturity, particularly if they are found to be unprofitable. Frequent or continuing temper tantrums may mean that the parents haven't learnt how to handle them. The first step is to prevent them. Does your child have adequate opportunity to burn up his energy by playing freely both outdoors and indoors without continual restrictions? Is your child being asked to make too many decisions at an age when he's not mature enough to do so, instead of just receiving a clear indication of what he is to do? Remember also that children between two and three are often going through a negative phase, when the answer to everything is 'no', whether they

Getting up should not be allowed to pay off as an adventure or as a pleasurable experience
▼▼▼

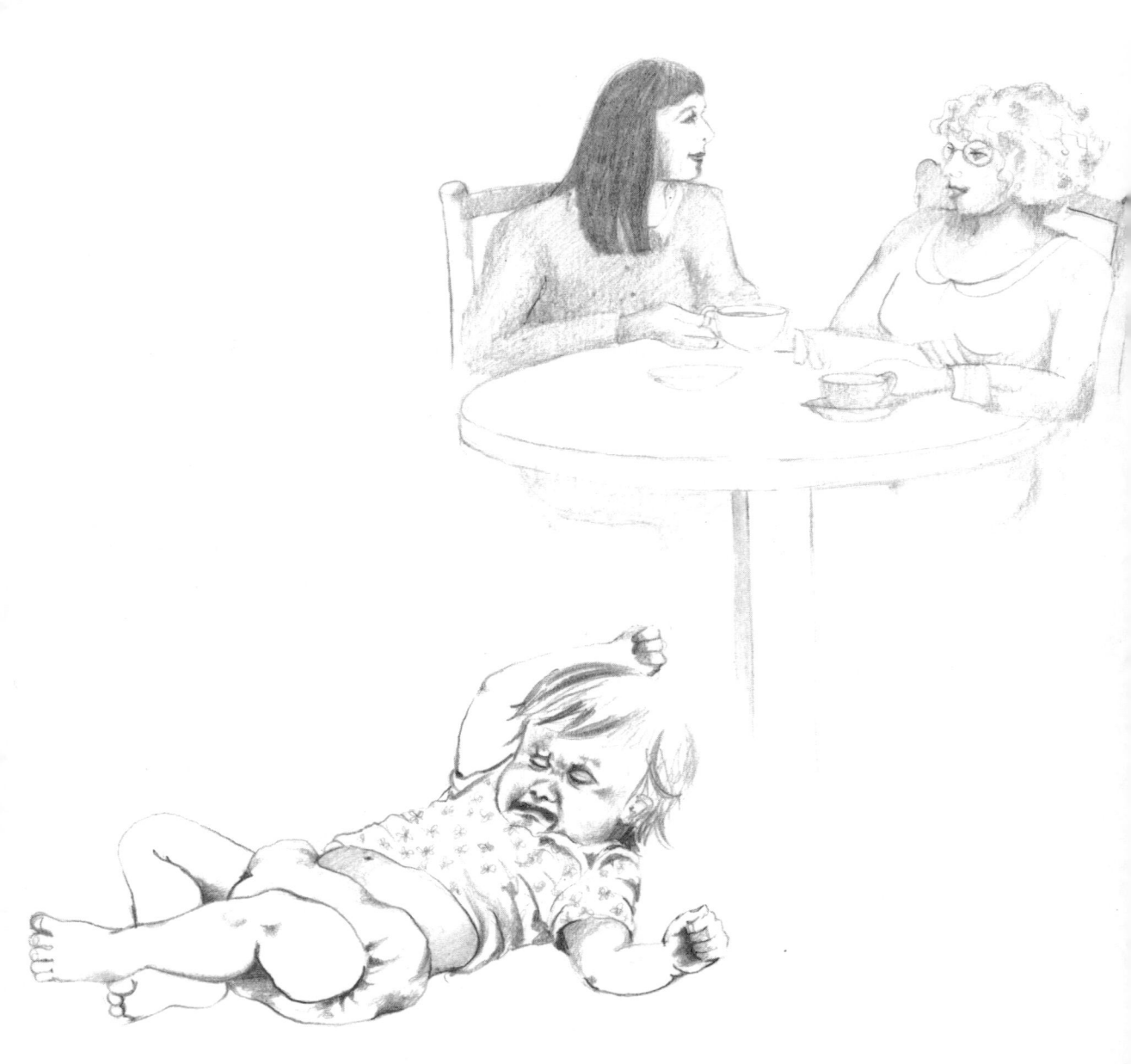

want to do it or not. Parents have to understand this and go along with it to some extent. Let him try to dress and undress himself and let him start to try feeding himself if he wants to.

A temper tantrum once in a while doesn't mean anything. You can't avoid them all. No parent has enough patience or time for that!

The best way of handling the occasional temper tantrum is to ignore it. Like the professional agitator, there is no point in performing without an audience. If it persists, don't get angry yourself, put him in a room and tell him he can come out when he wants to behave. If he starts having a temper tantrum in that room, ignore it. It's a way of gaining your attention and the last thing you want your child to learn is that tantrums pay off. Once he has cooled down, a quick sympathetic cuddle will usually promptly restore mutual affection.

Even these days, many parents, often as a result of their own childhood experience, think that children have to be spanked to be disciplined. True, spanking is one form of discipline, but it is one of the least effective. The word discipline means teaching; teaching your child by your own example of love and consistency, teaching them by what you say and encouraging them and praising them for the efforts they make rather than criticising them. One of the problems associated with hitting children as a form of discipline is that it teaches them that conflicts and problems can be resolved by violence, such as by hitting others. This is a lesson it's better that your child does not learn. Physical punishment should be at the bottom of your list of discipline techniques and it's best not to use it at all.

Head banging and breath holding

Repetitive banging of the head sometimes occurs during temper tantrums, sometimes implying an even more intense degree of anger and frustration. Breath holding is also a form of temper tantrum that occurs in some young babies who get so furiously angry that when they cry they hold their breath, turn blue and occasionally lose consciousness for a brief period. Although this is naturally very frightening for parents, it never causes any serious harm. However, in order to reassure yourself that there is nothing seriously wrong, it's wise to let your doctor know so that a careful check of your child will rule out any underlying problem.

Pica

Pica is the name given to the repeated seeking out and eating of substances other than food, such as paper, dirt, paint, hair and so on. If this type of behaviour persists, it may be the child's response to some sort of emotional stress or anxiety. This usually warrants consultation with a paediatrician or a specialist in child psychiatry. However most little explorers when outside will want to taste something as interesting as dirt or the occasional snail, and this doesn't necessarily mean there is an emotional crisis occurring.

Bad language

Four- and five-year-olds often go through a phase of 'dirty words'. They may not know what the words mean but they often realise they are being naughty and soon learn what an effect these words can have on an adult who hears them issuing from the mouth of a young 'innocent'. Usually the

> *Physical punishment should be at the bottom of your list of discipline techniques and it's best not to use it at all*
> ▼▼▼

'swear words' consist of lavatory terms, but if they hear their parents swear, they will certainly include those words too. If you are shocked or upset by these words emerging from your dear little angel, don't show it — this is the object of the exercise. Make it quite clear that you don't like to hear those words and you don't want them to use them. Ignoring them is the best technique, as well as teaching by your own example. The same approach applies to other antisocial habits, such as biting and kicking. All of these habits tend to be transient if handled sensibly.

JEALOUSY AND RIVALRY

Very often when a new baby comes along an older sister or brother is in the toddler age group. Most parents worry about whether the toddler will be jealous of the new arrival. You can take steps to anticipate and avoid this. It's important for your toddler to know well ahead of time that he is going to have a baby brother or sister, so that he can gradually get used to the idea. It's helpful for him to understand that the baby is growing inside his mother and to feel it move. He should be shown the preparations that are being made for the new baby and be allowed to help with them. Remember that there is going to be a period of separation while Mum is in hospital with the new baby, and the toddler should be prepared for this. He should be left in the care of whoever is going to be looking after him during this time for short periods before Mum goes to hospital. He will then not feel deserted because he is already secure in the knowledge that Mum will be coming back again.

When Mum comes home with the new baby, make sure that the toddler gets his share of mothering too. Make sure there is time to share his play and other activities while baby is asleep. Let him hold his new brother or sister if he wants to. He can sit in the middle of the bed, or on the floor or a soft carpet or blanket, without any risk to baby.

More mothers now participate in short stay or early discharge programs and while this helps normalise the birth process, it does result in mothers having to get back into household chores earlier. Planning some rest periods is very important. It may also present opportunities to have toddlers with you without the new baby.

SPEECH PROBLEMS

Most children start with single words at around one year of age and by two have some simple sentences. At this stage they may also chatter away in a totally incomprehensible language of their own. Some parents are worried about this, not realising that it's a perfectly normal stage

> *It's important for your toddler to know well ahead of time that he is going to have a baby brother or sister*
> ▼▼▼

of speech development. Speech becomes more and more intelligible during the next year. Sentences become longer and the child is capable of remembering short songs and nursery rhymes.

There are a number of reasons why speech may be delayed or clumsy, but if by the age of four other children obviously have difficulty in understanding your child, you should seek expert advice. Most parents are concerned that slow talking may mean slow mental development. It's certainly true that children who are developmentally delayed for any reason will be slow to talk, but they will also be slow in passing other milestones, such as sitting up, walking and feeding themselves. There is a wide variation in the normal range and the great majority of late talkers have normal intelligence. In some cases children have speech delay because they don't receive enough language stimulation, such as by having their parents talk with them often. The absence of other children in the family or friends' and neighbours' children in their own age group can also mean that they are receiving less stimulation to develop their own speech. Regular association with other children in a kindergarten will sometimes work wonders.

If your child has a hearing defect, this will usually delay speech development, so it is important for children with speech delay to have their hearing accurately tested.

All toddlers start by mispronouncing most of the words they use, but some continue to have special difficulty with one particular sound or another. This is not usually of any particular importance and corrects itself in time. However, if obvious speech problems continue after your child goes to school, seek expert advice Management will probably include speech therapy.

Sometimes children revert to baby talk after they have learnt to speak quite well. There is usually an obvious reason for this, such as the arrival of a new baby in the family, or some other stress, such as illness which may require admission to hospital. This is only a minor manifestation of insecurity and will usually promptly respond to a little extra care, affection and attention.

Tongue tie

Sometimes the fold of skin that joins the bottom of the tongue to the floor of the mouth is unduly prominent, but only very occasionally does it interfere with the free movement of the tongue and it rarely interferes with speech production. It usually corrects itself spontaneously as the tongue grows longer. If in doubt, consult your doctor.

If obvious speech problems continue after your child goes to school, seek expert advice

▼▼▼

Some children masturbate as a self-comforting habit just as others resort to thumb sucking ▼▼▼

STUTTERING

Stuttering is quite common between two and four when children are learning to form sentences and rapidly increasing their vocabulary. For most children it's only a passing phase and the great majority of children outgrow it within a few months. However, occasionally stuttering persists. It has a tendency to run in families and is more common in boys than girls. In children with a persistent stutter it's more obvious when they are upset or excited. If stuttering persists in the school-age child to an extent that it's obviously embarrassing for the child, it's wise to seek expert advice.

NAIL BITING

Nail biting is extremely common. About two-thirds of all children bite their nails although half of these will stop after a few years. Although in some children it reflects inner tension, in others there appears to be no obvious reason for the habit. Like thumb sucking, it disturbs parents, not children. It's a mistake to nag or punish a child for nail biting, and painting bitter substances on the nails does little good. It sometimes helps to keep the nails cut short, and with young girls an appeal to their vanity by giving them a manicure set for a present may do the trick. It's always worth thinking over whether your child is under any particular strain. Is there any undue pressure at school? Are you expecting too much of your child? Is there too much correction or punishment?

SEXUAL AWARENESS

In infants sexual awareness is merely part of their normal curiosity about their own bodies. They discover their genitals in just the same way that they discover their fingers or toes, their nose or their ears. By the time they are three they have developed an awareness of the difference between themselves and the opposite sex. At this age they also realise that handling or stimulating the genital area can produce pleasurable sensations. They continue to do this for two reasons: firstly, they obviously derive pleasure from it, secondly, it can be a form of reassurance when they are anxious. Some children masturbate as a self-comforting habit just as others resort to thumb sucking. This is not harmful, but excessive masturbation may be an indication that the child is exposed to stresses that he is finding hard to tolerate.

Virtually all children continue with some form of sex play when they are alone and in bed. It should only be a matter of concern if it is excessive or carried out in public or if it involves other children. Under these circumstances it's wise to seek expert advice. Never tell your child that sex play can cause sickness, or any harm, or that it's wicked. Such comments may have far-reaching consequences and subsequently interfere with a normal adjustment to adult sexual activities.

As well as being curious about their own genitals, children are also curious about those of other children. It's normal for them to want to satisfy their curiosity and the obvious way to do this is by having a look. There's nothing wrong with this but you should teach your child that this behaviour, while interesting, is not acceptable if done regularly. However, punishing a child for normal sexual exploratory behaviour may lead the child to believe that there is something bad about sex and may even elevate the level of curiosity so that the behaviour occurs more often.

BED-WETTING

It's rare for this to be due to a physical abnormality. It's also uncommon for bed-wetting alone to result from psychological disturbance although many children who are emotionally disturbed have a variety of symptoms which may include bed-wetting. Nearly half of all four-year-old boys still wet the bed at times. Little girls seem to achieve full bladder control somewhat earlier.

There are a number of factors concerned with bed-wetting. The main one seems to be the considerable variation in the time that children take to develop bladder control at night.

Sometimes a child who has been 'dry' for several months starts to wet the bed again. Occasionally this is due to a bladder infection and you should have this checked by your doctor. However, much more frequently it's related to some stress or anxiety which has caused the child to revert to a more immature pattern of behaviour. Bed-wetting doesn't need any treatment under the age of six years. If it continues after this, it's wise to consult your doctor and, if the condition persists, to seek the assistance of a paediatrician. A child may respond to simple measures, such as limiting fluid intake late in the day and/or rousing the child to pass urine when you go to bed. Your doctor will carry out a few simple checks to make sure there is no evidence of infection of the urine or any physical abnormality, although this is rarely the case. Treatment with medication is sometimes helpful, but the most effective method is the use of a battery powered alarm that rings and wakes the child as soon as the bed-wetting commences. This method should only be used under appropriate medical supervision.

Nearly half of all four-year-old boys still wet the bed at times
▼▼▼

Growing up

CHAPTER 6

Children and Play

Children live and learn by playing. Often adults fail to recognise the importance of play to children. As adults, our work and our leisure activities depend upon basic skills we learnt as children; to hold a pencil, write, read and express ourselves.

These basic skills or abilities are things we learnt in play. As we played we tried out different things to see what would happen and we looked for new ideas, all the while we were learning through play. We all know the pleasure the young child gains from playing with pots and saucepans and it can be seen how she learns from what she sees, feels and hears. She learns about shapes and sizes as she makes the discovery that the big object won't fit into the smaller one.

Questions are linked with play and a great deal of patience is required for parents to keep their child's curiosity satisfied. Play teaches a child to socialise, to share and communicate with others. Playing with other children is a necessary part of growing. The child who is deprived of early contact with other children may find it difficult to establish comfortable relation-ships outside the family later.

By playing, the child learns to work happily with others and also to resolve conflicts satisfactorily. Sometimes parents worry when children begin to fight, but it's reasonable to allow children to sort out their own differences without interference, unless someone is likely to be hurt or one child is always on the losing side. The fascinating thing about play is that, although it's so important for learning, it's still the child's own creation and is something that she enjoys.

Play material

It's not necessary to buy expensive or elaborate toys for a child. There can be great satisfaction in playing with simple, easily obtainable materials; for instance, large cardboard cartons make exciting cubbyhouses. They can be decorated with finger painting or papered with pictures from magazines. For the toddler, pots and pans from the kitchen cupboard are usually even more attractive than building blocks and beakers. As children get a little older, ordinary wooden boxes or large cardboard cartons make wonderful boats, dolls' beds or cars.

A child loves being able to play with natural materials, such as sand, water, clay or mud. If possible, arrange an area in the backyard as a sandpit where she can make a mess if she wants to. If you are going to provide her with a small wading pool or splash bath, make sure she only uses it under supervision and that it's emptied immediately after use.

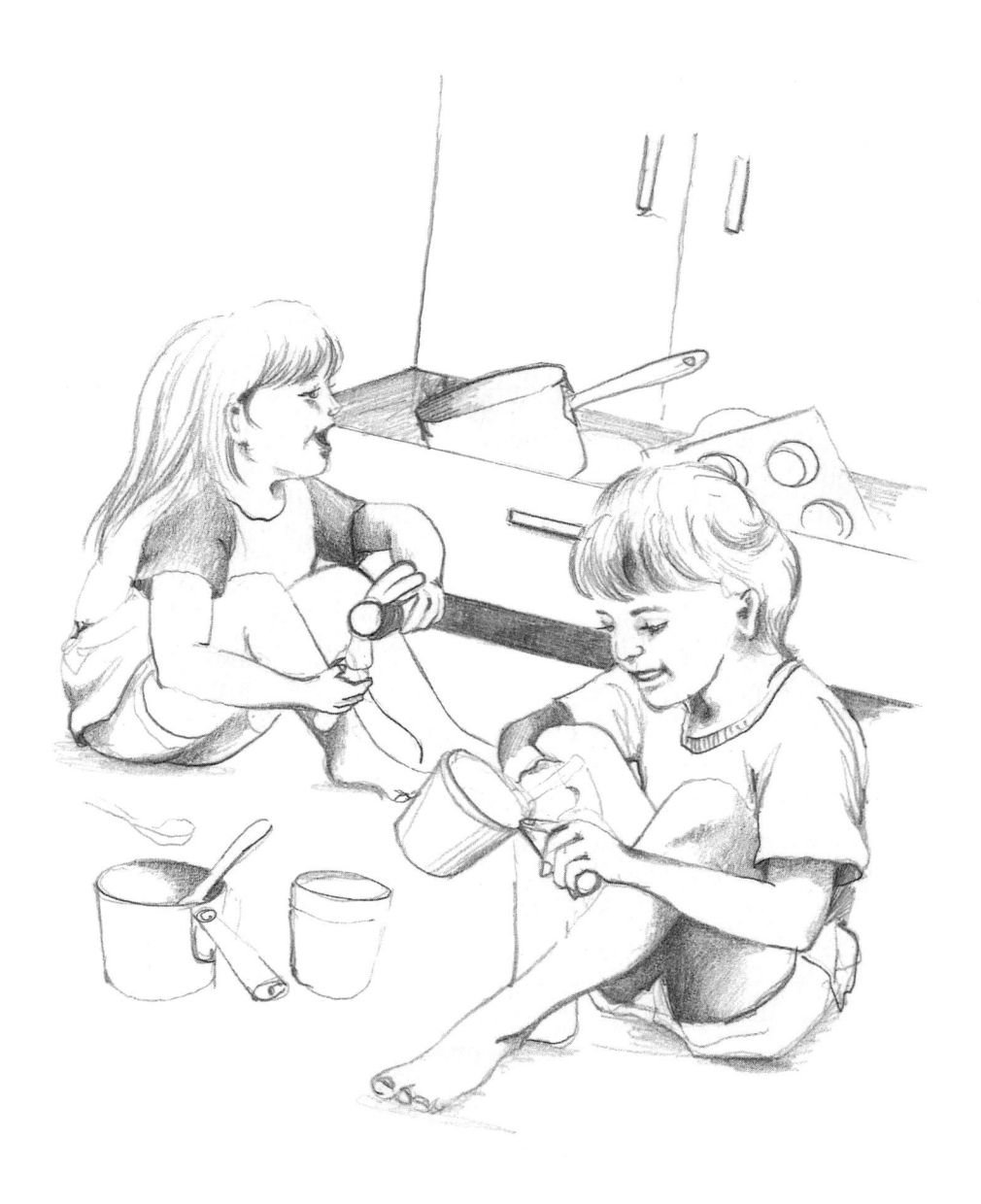

As children grow, play becomes more noisy and excited and you need to be prepared to accept this. If you are able to provide a playroom or rumpus room it gives the children all the scope they need and is certainly easier on Mum and Dad. In any case, there should be a toy box and they should learn, at an early age, the importance of tidying up when playtime is over.

As children grow, play becomes more noisy and excited and you need to be prepared to accept this ▼▼▼

Play and social development

Play helps the development of skills. From a very early age, baby will watch a mobile, beads or a rattle strung across her bassinette. First she'll watch and learn to fix on them with her eyes. Soon she'll begin to stretch out for them and in this way she'll learn to co-ordinate her hand and eye movements.

As children become mobile, they love to push or pull things. Simple things are best. Blocks on wheels with homes for pegs are a favourite, and the softness and comfort of rag dolls and soft woolly toys is often appealing. Toddlers like to imitate their parents and can often try to copy from them as they do their household chores. Let them help by all means, but remember they are very imitative at this age and require constant supervision. A little later, their imagination makes them more creative and their play activities become more complex. This is a time for cars, dolls and above all, blocks. Big blocks that they can use to build houses, castles, ships and trains are best.

Playing with other children

Children start by playing very happily by themselves. The most they want from an adult is a little diversion from time to time such as putting another toy within reach or putting a nest of blocks back together so they can undo them again. They certainly don't want to do things the way Mum or Dad thinks best. If a father who had wanted but did not get a train or a construction set as a child produces one for his three- or four-year-old, he's in for a surprise if he thinks his ideas as to how it should be used will be the same as those of his child. At this age, a simple wooden train with carriages that hook together is much more satisfying than an elaborate electric train.

Children begin to play with each other between the ages of one and two but at this age, although they are together, they tend to play individually. They take what they want from each other without ceremony and, if any attempt is made to take it from them, they either hang on to it grimly or, alternatively, take aggressive action, often to the embarrassment of their parents. Remember that if your two-year-old doesn't graciously give up her toys to a little visitor, she is behaving quite normally. Do not expect a child under the age of three to begin to understand about sharing things.

BOOKS AND STORIES

Introducing children to the fascinating world of books can start quite early. Begin around one year of age with rag books that will not tear, and graduate to books with thick, hard to tear pages and with large coloured pictures that the child can easily recognise and identify. By two years, the child is eager for stories. At first, these need to be short, as her concentration is limited. She will want to hear her favourite story over and over again. If there's a new baby brother or sister by this time, it's often helpful to sit your toddler down next to you while you're feeding the baby and tell her one of her favourite stories. Remember that for children up to five or six years, it is difficult to separate fact from fiction. Father Christmas and fairies are, and should be, very real for the toddler, otherwise they miss a wonderful experience. At the end of this chapter, there is a list of toys for children of different ages and a suitable list of books. We hope they are already familiar to you, but if not, you and your children will enjoy the experience of discovering them.

TELEVISION

A child can learn a lot from television, but there are also programs that are not suitable for children. Used wisely, general knowledge can be expanded, but a check should always be made on what the child is learning. Selected viewing is advisable, with a limit on watching times so that television is only a small part of a child's pleasure time and does not fill it all. You may notice that after a child has had a long spell in front of the television set she may be irritable, aggressive or very active. Children often need to let off steam after watching television. A good rule of thumb for children under primary school age is to limit selected viewing to about one hour each day.

PETS

Animals love children and children love animals. Birds and fish have little to offer the very young and some breeds of cats tend to be rather independent, but a child and her dog can become inseparable companions. Do remember, though, that kittens and puppies grow up!

Children often need to let off steam after watching television
▼▼▼

Children and play 71

Suggestions for Play and Toys at Different Ages

The first year

In the first twelve months play will centre around physical contact with Mum and Dad who need to be aware of each stage of development and so be ready to help the baby master these. Rolling, sitting, crawling and standing can be encouraged through play. She will need objects which are easy to grasp, brightly coloured, or make a sound, strong enough to withstand being bitten or dropped, not so small they can be swallowed, and above all they need to be easily washable.

Birth to six months

- Rattles of a single bright colour, light but strong, washable and unbreakable.
- Strong, large, wooden beads, or rings strung across the cot.
- A brightly coloured mobile attached to the cot.
- Strong, soft, chewable plastic toys: washable and unbreakable.

Six to twelve months

- A large playpen, preferably with a floor. Make sure that it's designed so that she cannot catch fingers or toes, there are no sharp angles or corners, and that she cannot get her head between the bars.
- Large, brightly coloured balls. Soft, washable ones that she can grasp are the best.
- A teddy bear or a rag doll can be introduced at this stage: soft dolls are much better than ones made of hard plastic.
- Squeaky play animals without removable parts.
- Empty cardboard containers with lids to put on and take off.
- Floating bath toys.

One to two years

- Nests of hollow blocks or beakers.
- A sandpit with a bucket and spade.
- Empty plastic ice-cream cartons to play with in the sandpit or to take to the beach.
- Wooden trains or cars to push or pull, but make sure the wheels are too big to swallow if they come off.
- A peg board with coloured pegs.
- A few rag books with brightly coloured pictures.
- Saucepans and their lids and pans with a wooden spoon.
- Blocks.
- Soft dolls are still popular at this age.

Two to four years

- Large wooden blocks — you can make these very cheaply

Mum and Dad need to be aware of each stage of development and so be ready to help the baby master these
▼▼▼

yourself from scraps of hardwood. Make sure they are smooth and don't have splinters.
- Simple puzzles and felt building sets.
- A tricycle: make sure it's not too big for the child. It's better to start with dinkies or push along toys.
- Simple sturdy picture books with bright pictures.
- Crayons and paper, but ensure the colour in the crayon is not poisonous. Use crayons that are labelled non-toxic.
- Finger painting or brush painting using water soluble non-toxic poster paints.
- Plasticine and clay can also be used in this way.
- Dolls for dressing and undressing.
- Puppets and cuddly toys.
- By now she should have a toy box and be starting to learn to put toys away after play.
- If she has a playroom or rumpus room, put a blackboard or drawing board on one wall.
- Old clothes for dressing up are always popular.
- In the yard there should be a sandpit and perhaps a tyre swing.
- As your child gets older you will be able to introduce bats and balls, skipping ropes and other toys.

READING LIST

This list has been supplied by Shearers Young People's Bookshop at Gordon in Sydney. The books are available there or at other bookstores catering for children.

This list of course reflects our personal tastes to some extent and is not intended to be complete — there are many other suitable books for children available. Don't forget the children's section of your local public library.

Music and poetry are also important cultural activities that should be encouraged. There are many records and cassette tapes available that are specially designed for children to encourage and develop an interest in music and the arts.

Puppets and marionettes of various types and puppet theatres are also a good way of encouraging an interest in the arts. They frequently appear on children's programs on television.

FOR TODDLERS

Start with board and cloth books — sturdy, hard to tear, brightly coloured books which will be mostly pictures, for this age group.

BOOKS TO READ TO TODDLERS

Counting, ABC alphabet and picture books
Books about animals —

Reading, music, poetry and theatre should be all encouraged
▼▼▼

Children and play 73

include some about Australian birds and animals

Books about nature, everyday life and children's adventures

Books about transport, travel and machinery

Fairy stories for fun and fantasy

For children four to seven

Gradually introduce books they can begin to read for themselves.

A Book for Me to Read — Ainsworth series
Let's Read and Find Out series
Ladybird books
Read to Yourself books
Ready to Read series
Golden Books — for example, *Scuffy the Tugboat* and *Tottle the Train*
Beginner Books and other Dr Seuss books

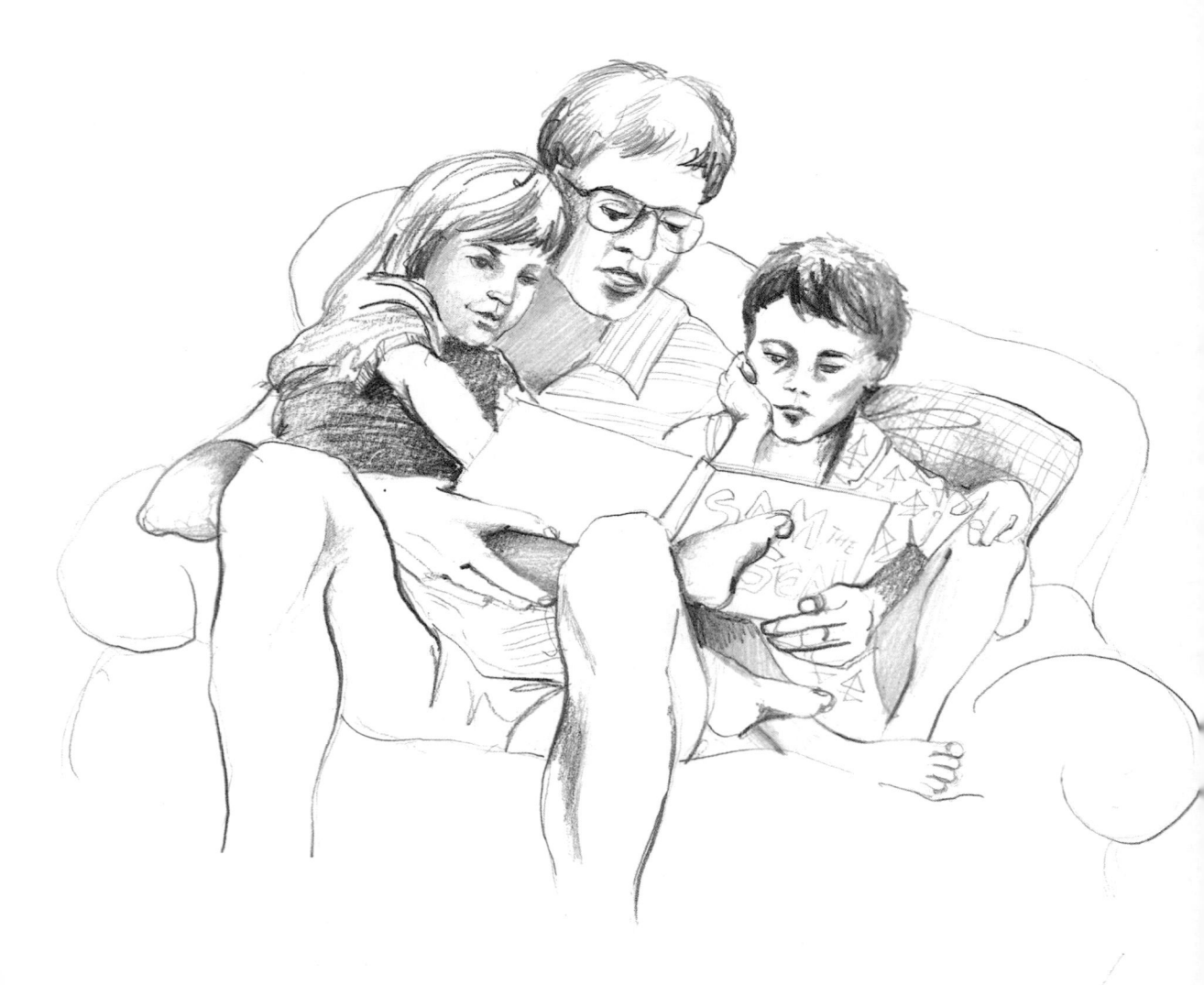

For children of all ages

Hans Christian Andersen's fairytales
Grimm's fairytales
Robert Louis Stevenson, *A Child's Garden of Verse*
J. M. Barrie, *Peter Pan*
A. A. Milne, Winnie the Pooh series
Beatrix Potter, *The Tale of Peter Rabbit* (and other books)
Rudyard Kipling, *Just So Stories*
Kenneth Graham, *The Wind in the Willows*
Lewis Carroll, *Alice in Wonderland*
Ludwig Bemelmans, *Madeline*

Books about Australia

May Gibbs, *Snugglepot and Cuddlepie*
Norman Lindsay, *The Magic Pudding*
Ivan Southall, *Hill's End* (and other books)
Leslie Rees, *Shy the Platypus* (and other books)
Colin Thiele, *Storm Boy*
Dick Roughsey, *The Rainbow Serpent*

Play and the sick child

Fortunately, the majority of children's illnesses only last a few days. However, if they are potentially more serious, they are likely to be treated in hospital. If your child is unfortunate enough to suffer a more prolonged illness at home, a few simple words of advice may help.

Unlike an adult, young children cannot occupy their time reading and the younger they are, the shorter their attention span will be. Simple games and activities that they can master without undue physical or mental effort will be the most popular. For many of these you will need a wide flat tray. A bed tray with folding legs is a useful acquisition, but a flat board supported on a chair each side of the bed is equally effective. When a child is sick, her play interests will change and at first she is more likely to want familiar objects such as her teddy bear or to have Mum or Dad read to her or tell her stories. If she is confined to bed for a lengthy period it may be possible for her to spend part of the day on a lounge. This will give her a change of scene and allow the bed to air and be made up. This could also coincide with a suitable television program, appropriate for her age, but it's wise to avoid making prolonged television viewing a substitute for

Simple games and activites are best for a child who is sick in bed
▼▼▼

more formative play stimulation and proper rest periods.

It may be helpful to divide the day into sections so that she can have some time with messy play, such as dough and finger painting, some constructional playtime using blocks and building toys, some time for table games with Mum, brothers, sisters or friends, and some reading time.

One of her main needs will be to have Mum or Dad with her, so try to arrange to do some household chores in her room or while she's lying down on the lounge.

Family and friends may want to bring her toys. If so, suggest they look particularly for toys that give her an opportunity to use her imagination. There is only a limited scope for pull along toys, trucks and trains for the child in bed, but building sets, colouring-in books, plasticine, crayons and cut-outs can provide interesting occupation for hours. It's sensible to give only one new toy at a time. Remember also that, with a little imagination, many play activities can be manufactured on the spot, such as sewing, cutting pictures out of old magazines and making scrap books.

As convalescence proceeds, try to lead her more and more back into normal activities. It's only natural that she should expect and receive special consideration and attention while she is sick, but she should realise that it's not reasonable for this to continue once she is well again.

PLAY AND THE HANDICAPPED CHILD

Play activities are a very important way of providing appropriate stimulation for children with physical or mental handicaps. It must be borne in mind that they will have difficulty in keeping up with other children and that their play activities will need to be tailored to fit in with their handicap.

All children learn by what they experience through their senses, and a handicapped child also needs stimulation through seeing, hearing, touching and smelling. It provides an opportunity to give her much needed contact with those of her own age group or peer group and to teach her to join in play with others. In the case of children with orthopaedic problems who require exercises to improve the function, strength and range of movement of their limbs, it's often possible to introduce these in the form of play activities.

There are a number of special schools available for children who, for various reasons, are unable to take their place in a normal class. In addition, a number of schools have special

Building sets, colouring books, plasticine, crayons and cut-outs can provide interesting occupation for hours
▼▼▼

classes or have remedial teachers present for children who require special attention. The preferred model is to provide for the special needs of individual children in normal schools, even if it means a separate class.

Your paediatrician and teacher, with the assistance of a paediatric social worker, can advise you about the most appropriate way of dealing with your child's particular problem.

All children learn by what they experience through their senses
▼▼▼

CHAPTER 7

HANDICAPPED CHILDREN

Most expectant parents have an unconscious mental image of what their baby will be like. This is usually the image of a healthy, perfectly formed baby. It's also normal for parents to have some fears during pregnancy that their baby might be handicapped.

When they are born, many babies don't fit the idealised picture. They may be premature, a different sex from the one wanted or have other minor problems in the first few days of life. But in spite of initial disappointments, the mental image and the reality soon become reconciled with each other and a firm bond is established between parents and baby.

However, the initial feelings of despair may be devastating when the baby is born with a serious handicap. Parents of handicapped children first learn of the problem in various ways. They may suddenly discover or be told about the child's handicap soon after birth, or, in less obvious cases, the realisation may only slowly dawn upon them. It's normal to feel disappointed and let down, and to experience a variety of emotions. These may include feeling guilty, denying there is a problem at all, being angry with the doctors in the hospital, being resentful, feeling helpless and overwhelmed, and searching for a miracle cure or another opinion which will say everything is all right. These emotional phases may take different times to pass for different people. The final stage is coming to a realistic acceptance of the handicap so that the family can then work together with the co-operation of professionals to help their baby achieve his full potential. It's worth stressing one further point. If you are seriously concerned that your child is not responding to stimuli in the way that your friends' children are at a comparable age, or if he appears to be falling behind as other children progress, it's better to discuss your worries with your family doctor and to get him to refer you, if necessary, to an appropriate paediatrician, rather than to continue to live with the torment of ignorance, fear, anxiety and guilt.

A team approach is needed to help the handicapped child. The team may include doctors, nurses, psychologists, social workers, speech pathologists, physiotherapists, occupational therapists, teachers and, of course, both parents.

Physical Handicaps

In some ways it's easier for parents to accept physical handicaps than mental handicaps. At least other people can see what's wrong and therefore be more understanding. In our society, physical handicaps often don't have the social stigma that some people still feel about mental or intellectual handicaps.

Despite these feelings, the problems that face children with physical handicaps are just as real as those facing the mentally handicapped.

Deafness

It may take some time to recognise that your baby is deaf, even if his hearing is profoundly impaired. If he doesn't seem to respond to sound, particularly if the noise is loud and close to him, when a baby with normal hearing would be expected to start to cry, you should get your doctor to test his hearing. There are now ways of testing even small babies and a 'wait and see' policy is no longer acceptable. Early diagnosis is important so that the baby may be encouraged to use his other senses for learning from an early age. The early stimulation of the deaf infant, using his other senses, helps him to experience what the world about him is like. The important thing is to find out rather than hope that it will get better.

Hand in hand with the ability to hear sounds goes the development of speech. There are many causes of delayed or defective speech but one of the most important is impaired hearing. From the cooing and babbling noises that baby makes comes the gradual development of intelligible words, first single syllables and then short sentences and gradually longer and longer words and strings of words. But if there is no effective input of sound there is no stimulus to produce speech. Some of the problems that the parent of a profoundly deaf child has to face are well expressed in the following letter.

'Megan was born totally deaf. She has no speech and hears nothing, even with the most powerful hearing aids.

'To get Megan's attention I have to move within her field of vision and attract her attention by waving, touching her, banging the floor so she can feel the vibrations or flashing the lights.

'I cannot call Megan to tell her which room I am in; I have to go and tell her. If she wants me she has to look in every part of the house until she finds me; she cannot use sound clues or call me.

'Megan has many medical appointments. This interferes with her life as well as that of the rest of the family and my working life.

The problems that face children with physical handicaps are just as real as those facing the mentally handicapped
▼▼▼

Handicapped children 79

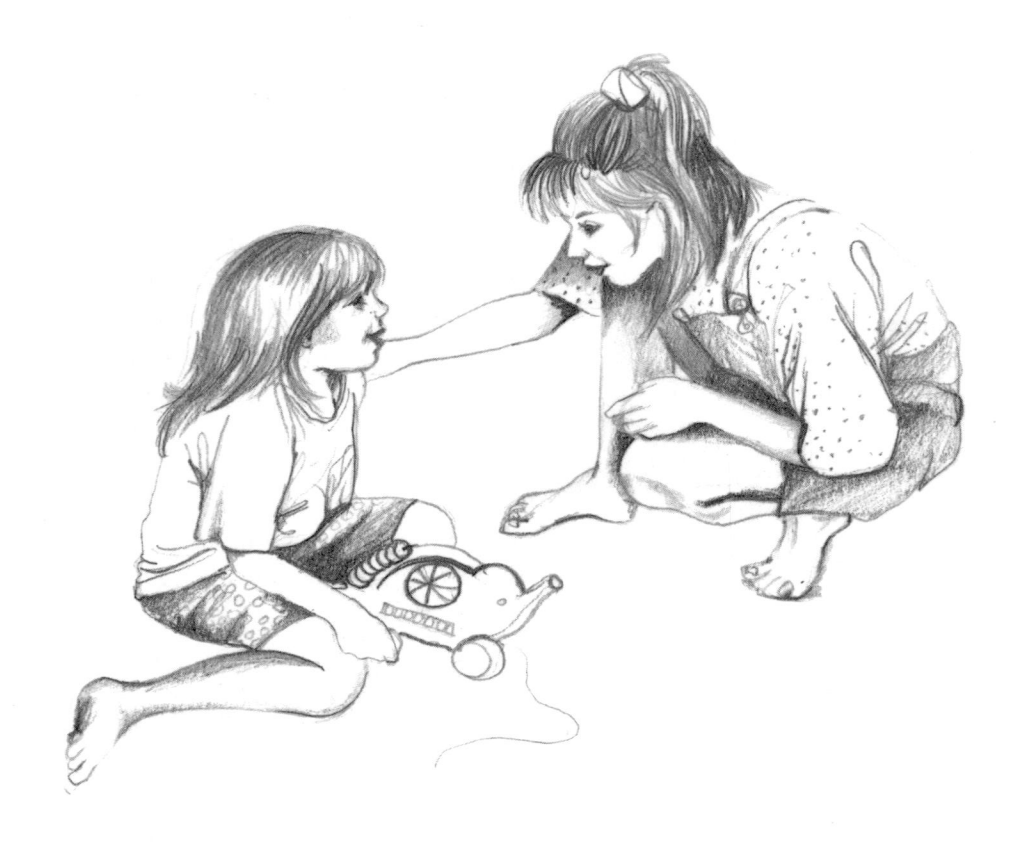

'Megan's deafness makes her paticularly vulnerable. She cannot hear traffic or any noises that a hearing child would know indicate danger and one must always remember that, if there is any urgent threat to her safety, one cannot call out to attract her attention and warn her.'

Megan and her family are learning sign language. It takes years to reach a standard adequate to communicate all the things one would be able to teach, advise, discuss, explain to a hearing child. Thus everyday subjects, such as whether she would like a drink or something to eat, what she wants to play with, where the family is going, who people are, whether things are hot or cold, all take much longer to explain. More complicated issues, often relating to safety, are extremely difficult and sometimes impossible to communicate.

Parents of deaf children, as

well as the child himself, need expert guidance by a trained teacher of the deaf so that the child may be encouraged by every possible means to talk and to develop language. If there is some residual hearing, a hearing aid will be useful but it must be realised that these devices are not selective and can cause exaggeration of environmental and background noises that may interfere with comprehension of the spoken word.

Cochlear implantation is now being offered in younger and younger infants and the early results are encouraging for both hearing and speech.

Many moderately deaf children can attend a normal school but profoundly deaf children require special educational facilities.

Blindness

Blindess is much less common than deafness. Severe deafness, sufficient to require special schooling, occurs in one in every thousand children while blindness or markedly impaired vision has an incidence of only one in 2500 children.

Most blind children have some vision, even if it is only the recognition of light and darkness. Blindness should be suspected if random and unco-ordinated eye movements persist after the age of six weeks. If baby does not start to look at you and follow your face with his eyes by the time he is three or four months of age, you should consult your doctor or take baby to your local hospital to have his sight checked.

Most causes of blindness in children cannot be cured. Parents of a blind child need expert and sympathetic advice from an early age. Preschool teachers are usually available from the various organisations oriented to blind children.

Common eye problems such as squint and abnormalities of vision are discussed in a later chapter.

Delayed Development

A child with a developmental disability will learn to do new things, but this will be at his own individual pace. He will be slower than average with all his milestones and achievements. The development of skills, such as sitting, walking, understanding words, speaking and toilet training will be delayed or may not even be achieved. As developmental delay may vary from mild to profound, the slowness of achievement will vary accordingly. The milder the degree of delay, the less obvious it will be, and milder causes may not be recognised for some years.

There are many causes of developmental disability. In only

A child with a developmental disability will learn to do new things at his own individual pace
▼▼▼

Home and clinic counselling is available to help developmentally disabled children and their families ▼▼▼

a small percentage is there any risk of it happening again in the family. In some cases it's due to some form of birth injury or lack of oxygen during the birth process, but often the abnormality has occurred during development of the baby. Sometimes it's due to an infection occurring early in pregnancy, such as rubella. Occasionally meningitis, encephalitis and serious head injuries may cause permanent brain damage, but it's important to realise that full recovery may often follow these conditions. In very many cases, no cause can be found.

DOWN'S SYNDROME

This condition is usually able to be recognised shortly after birth by an experienced paediatrician or nurse. Even when the diagnosis appears certain, it should always be confirmed by examining and counting the chromosomes in the baby's blood cells — a test which takes about a week. Children with Down's syndrome always have some degree of developmental disability but some are less severely affected than others. There is also a higher than normal incidence of other major abnormalities, such as congenital heart disease and bowel obstruction. While babies with Down's syndrome obviously differ from other children, they are generally affectionate, loving and usually fit in without much trouble to most families while they are young.

Down's syndrome occurs more commonly when the mother is over thirty-five years of age. It's possible to make the diagnosis from fluid collected from the womb at about fourteen weeks of pregnancy (amniocentesis) or earlier by a sample or biopsy of the placenta (chorionic villus sampling) so that the option of terminating the pregnancy can be considered by the parents.

MANAGEMENT OF DEVELOPMENTAL DISABILITY

Early advice and support is important, but planning for the management of the disability starts with an assessment and evaluation of the extent of the disability and its possible causes. It must also include appropriate counselling of the family and ongoing support for the family both in the clinic and in the home. While the child's medical condition and evaluation is important, it is equally important to know the attitudes of the family and their ability to cope with this major family crisis. Different societies vary considerably in their attitude to disabled children.

Special clinics exist to help these children and their families and these can be found by talking to your family doctor or paediatrician. Home visiting is important in understanding the particular needs of an individual family.

Many early intervention programs have been proposed from time to time. Some are extremely supportive of families and result in children who achieve their full potential within a coping family. Others may result in children reaching milestones earlier but do not affect the final end point. It is difficult to generalise and families with these problems need to be given expert help and advice.

Accepting a handicap can be a long and difficult task. There is no right way for everyone nor is there a normal time frame in which all people reach the various milestones.

CHAPTER 8

THE SICK CHILD

Older children can tell you when they are not feeling well, but with a baby, you have to notice that there may be a problem. If your infant is listless, fretful, not eating or feels hot to touch, you could make a few simple checks. See if there is a skin rash or diarrhoea and check the temperature. It's quite easy to use a thermometer, but useful if on a visit to the baby clinic you are shown how to place it and read it.

If you are in any doubt as to the course of your child's illness, it's always safest to consult your doctor. You can also use your commonsense. The child who has lots of energy, runs around and eats well is unlikely to have a problem requiring immediate attention. On the other hand a baby who has a temperature, is drowsy and feeds poorly usually needs to see a doctor straightaway.

WHEN TO CALL A DOCTOR

When your child appears very sick and you feel that she needs immediate medical attention you can: call your own local doctor; call an ambulance to take the child to the casualty department of the nearest general hospital or children's hospital; if the problem is very urgent and you live close to a hospital, use your own car, but drive carefully. In urgent circumstances delay is your greatest enemy and you should therefore use the quickest, safest way to get a doctor to your child or your child to the doctor.

The following problems need prompt medical attention:

- Coma, convulsions, severe headache
- Excessive or unexpected bleeding
- Difficulty in breathing
- Changes in colour — paleness, blueness, mottling of the skin
- Persistent high temperature
- Shock, with poor pulses and cold clammy skin
- Severe pain
- Continued vomiting or diarrhoea (especially babies and infants)
- Unusual lumps, especially if tender or large
- Swallowed or inhaled objects, tablets or poisons
- Any major accident

Medicines

While tablets and medicines are necessary for some problems, often minor illnesses cure themselves without any medication at all. If your doctor prescribes medicine or tablets for your child, make sure you understand the instructions about how often to give it, how long to give it for, and how to store it. Don't be afraid to ask your doctor these questions. When giving your child the medicine, measure it accurately. Measuring glasses are much more accurate than teaspoons which vary considerably in size.

Antibiotics should only be given on medical advice and you should never give your child medicine or tablets that were prescribed for someone else. In fact most families unnecessarily store partially used medicines. When you have finished with medicines or tablets, get rid of them safely. All medicines and tablets should be kept out of reach of children, preferably in a cupboard with a childproof lock.

Fever

If your child has a high temperature you should, of course, consult your doctor. To reduce the temperature, sponge your child's body all over with lukewarm water. Don't wrap your child up in warm clothes as this will make the temperature climb higher. Your child will be more comfortable if completely exposed or covered with just a light sheet until the temperature starts to fall. Although she may not want to eat, offer fluids frequently. Fruit juices and water are the most popular. Jelly, lemonade or ice-cream will sometimes be taken when other foods are refused. It's best if the fruit juice and lemonade is diluted to half strength with water. Paracetamol (Panadol) in the correct dose can often help your child to sleep and reduce fever, and don't forget the value of cuddling and comfort — often the most effective remedy of all for a small child who is not feeling well.

Problems of the Ears, Nose and Throat

Coughs and colds

The common cold accounts for more than half of all illnesses seen in young children. The germ responsible for the common cold is a virus. Several different viruses are capable of causing colds, and this explains why some children can develop one cold after the other. Antibiotics have no effect on viruses, but the

Never give your child medicine or tablets that were prescribed for someone else
▼▼▼

natural body defences usually overcome them within a few days.

Parents are often worried that their children will catch colds by playing outside in cold weather, particularly if it's also wet. However, the most important factor is the spread of infection from one child to another by coughing and sneezing. This is the reason why colds and bronchitis are particularly common around the age of three to six years when your child first starts going to preschool or school and mixes with a number of other young children. A cough syrup may help your child to sleep at night but the traditional cough mixture is of little value apart from this.

CROUP

This is caused by a virus which causes some swelling in the upper airway, producing noisy breathing (stridor). It's often first noticed in the evening. As well as noisy breathing there may be a cough which sounds like the barking of a seal. There is no really effective treatment for croup that you can give at home and most mild causes improve by themselves. People used to believe that having the child breath moist air, such as by running a hot shower in the bathroom to fill it with steam, was beneficial. This probably does not help, but may be soothing.

If the noisy breathing becomes worse or if your child is looking more unwell, you should contact your doctor promptly or go to a hospital casualty department.

NOSE BLEEDS

These are very common in children and may be due to nose picking or can occur without any obvious reason. Firm compression of the lower soft part of the nostrils for five to ten minutes will usually control nose bleeding. An icepack applied to the bridge of the nose can sometimes be helpful, but compression of the nostrils is by far the most important thing to do. If the nose bleeding is severe and does not stop with these simple remedies, it's time to seek help from your doctor.

SORE THROATS, TONSILLITIS AND SWOLLEN GLANDS

There are many different kinds of throat infections, some due to viruses and some to bacteria. It's common to have a sore throat at the beginning of a cold. When the tonsils are infected, your child usually has a high fever and feels sick. Headache and vomiting may occur and swallowing is painful. The glands at the side of the neck often become swollen and tender. Occasionally, children with tonsillitis complain of stomach ache.

Cough syrup may help your child to sleep at night but is of little value apart from this ▼▼▼

Tonsillitis is often caused by a bacterial infection and usually requires prompt treatment with an antibiotic to overcome the infection and prevent complications. Penicillin does not normally affect the bacteria in the bowels but a broad acting antibiotic may lead to diarrhoea. Eating acidophilus based yoghurt may hasten recovery by helping to recolonise the bowels.

If the glands in the neck become swollen and tender, this is usually a result of infection entering via the tonsils. If the swollen glands persist, or increase in size, or if there is a continuing fever, consult your doctor.

TONSILS AND ADENOIDS

The tonsils and adenoids are composed of material called lymphoid tissue, or lymph glands. Lymph glands are also found in the neck, the armpits, the groin and inside the body. The purpose of this tissue is to help produce immunity to various diseases. This is part of the body's natural defence mechanism against infection.

While children are building up their immunity to various diseases the tonsils and other lymph glands become larger, until the age of seven or eight when they begin to decrease in size. Occasionally, the tonsils themselves become infected. Repeated infections of the tonsils, over a period of two years, is sometimes best treated by removal of the tonsils, although this is not done nearly as often as in the past.

Sometimes the tonsils become so large that they interfere with breathing, especially during sleep. This can be a reason for removing the tonsils in some cases.

Enlarged adenoids can sometimes interfere with breathing through the nose or cause recurrent ear infections, and this may be an indication for their removal, but not necessarily for removal of the tonsils at the same time. Children with enlarged adenoids usually snore and tend to breath with their mouths open.

MIDDLE EAR INFECTIONS (OTITIS MEDIA)

Acute middle ear infections are common in children from infancy up to about eight years of age. Affected babies cannot complain of pain but will be irritable, feverish and may pull at their ears or rub them. In older children there may be severe earache, often at night, associated with fever and sometimes vomiting. There may be an associated cold, bronchitis or one of the infectious diseases such as measles. The infection may also follow swimming in contaminated water. Your doctor can confirm middle ear infection by examination of the ear drums and will prescribe a suitable antibiotic. If the infection

Tonsils and adenoids are composed of material called lymphoid tissue, or lymph glands
▼▼▼

If a discharging ear persists there may be a progressive hearing loss
▼▼▼

is not detected early, the ear drum may perforate and the ear will discharge. If a discharging ear persists, or if there are repeated attacks of acute middle ear infection, there may be a progressive hearing loss, so it is important for ear infections to be properly treated and checked again later to make sure that recovery is complete.

GLUE EAR

Glue ear can affect children from the first year of life but is most common between three and six years of age. There is a persistent accumulation of thick fluid behind the ear drum (i.e. in the middle ear) which may cause repeated earache and partial hearing loss. The eustachian tube, which connects the middle ear to the back of the nose and throat, becomes blocked, and fluid which accumulates in the middle ear becomes thicker.

If the symptoms cause problems, particularly if there is hearing loss, ventilation tubes may be needed in the ears. The child is given a short general anaesthetic and, using a special operating ear microscope, a tiny plastic ventilation tube (grommet) is inserted into the ear drum. This tube acts as an artificial eustachian tube for six to nine months. With adequate and continued treatment, hearing is usually restored to normal.

OUTER EAR INFECTIONS (OTITIS EXTERNA)

Infections of the first part of the ear canal are quite common. They occur more often in the summer and are often associated with swimming. The ear may have a slight discharge and will often be itchy. They often respond to antibiotic ear drops.

WAX IN THE EARS

Wax is a protective substance produced by the ear canal. Wax which seeps into the outer part of the ear can be wiped away with a cotton bud or the tip of a handkerchief. There is never any need to insert anything into the ear to clean it. Occasionally the wax can become quite hard and accumulates in the ear canal. Wax softeners bought from the chemist will usually solve this problem although occasionally the wax may need to be syringed out by your doctor.

COMMON EYE PROBLEMS

Babies can see right from the time they are born. They are able to follow slowly moving objects held about 20 cm from them. However, it is not until five or six weeks that they start to follow slowly moving objects around the room. The colour of the eyes is determined by the amount of pigment deposited in the iris — the coloured portion of the eye around the central black pupil. This takes some time to occur. This is why all newborn babies have blue eyes which may gradually change in colour during the first year or so of life.

SQUINT (STRABISMUS)

Infants and young children may appear to be cross-eyed, especially if they have a broad, flat nose bridge. During the first six months of life, your baby's eyes may cross from time to time but as eye movements become better co-ordinated this should disappear. If a crossed eye is neglected, that eye will become lazy and the squint may become worse. If you suspect your child may have a squint, it's wise to seek early diagnosis and treatment. Treatment is usually commenced by covering the good eye to help the lazy one develop normal vision. Glasses may be necessary and eye exercises are useful in certain cases. An operation to align the eye muscles is sometimes necessary.

VISUAL PROBLEMS

Children may be short sighted, long sighted or have uneven curvature of the cornea; this is called astigmatism. Children will not usually be aware that they have poor vision but they may want to sit at the front of the class at school or hold things very close to their eyes. Glasses may be prescribed for this. Even very young children will wear glasses quite happily, if they are necessary.

WATERING AND DISCHARGING EYES

Babies are often born with watering or discharge from one or both eyes. If this persists, it's usually due to blockage of the tear duct. Most cases will respond to gentle massage right in the corner of the eye, several times each day. If watering persists after the age of six months, the blocked duct can be opened in a very simple operation, where a fine probe is passed into the duct to clear it.

CONJUNCTIVITIS AND STYES

Conjunctivitis causes redness and discharge from the eyes. It's usually due to infection with a bacteria or virus and generally involves both eyes. It usually responds very promptly to antibiotic eye drops and bathing.

A sty is a small boil due to inflammation at the base of one of the eyelashes. Bathing with warm water and the application of a local antibiotic ointment usually clears it up promptly. A red,

All newborn babies have blue eyes which may gradually change in colour during the first year of life

▼▼▼

The sick child 89

swollen eye suggests an eye infection and should be promptly seen by a doctor.

ITCHY EYES

Some children, especially those with allergies, will often rub their eyes and complain of itchiness. This is usually an allergic reaction to irritants in the air and is particularly common around springtime when there is a lot of pollen in the air, or after swimming in a heavily chlorinated pool.

EYE INJURIES

One of the most common eye injuries is a foreign particle lodging on the surface of the eyeball. The eye becomes red, irritable and waters freely. If you think something may have lodged in your child's eye, it's best to go to the doctor rather than attempt to remove it yourself.

If any chemical is accidentally spilt in the eye, the eye should be immediately washed by splashing lots of tap water into it and medical help should be sought without delay.

Blunt injury, such as may occur from a ball or a fist hitting the child in the eye, can cause various problems. Commonly a 'black eye' results, but bleeding can also occur internally into the eye, or the delicate cornea (the window through which we see) may be grazed. Sharp objects such as scissors or knives can lead to permanent loss of vision if the eyeball is penetrated. All eye injuries should be regarded seriously and your doctor must be consulted promptly.

COMMON SKIN PROBLEMS

The skin is a remarkable structure. Although a variety of organisms are present on its surface, unless it is broken it effectively protects the underlying tissue and organs from infection. It's also the most important means by which we regulate our body temperature. The energy necessary for muscle movement produces heat which is lost from the surface of the skin by evaporation. More vigorous exercise produces perspiration which is an even more effective method of getting rid of heat. Within the skin are fine, specialised nerve endings which allow us to appreciate pain, heat, cold, touch and pressure. Vitamin D is manufactured in the skin by the action of sunlight.

Throughout our lives, the skin is undergoing a continuing process of wear and replacement. As the protective outer layers are being slowly rubbed away, they are replaced. When skin loss occurs, as from a cut or a burn, this process of renewal is very

If you think something may have lodged in your child's eye, go to the doctor ▼▼▼

much accelerated. When an area of skin is completely destroyed, as by a deep burn, or when a cut passes right through the skin into the tissues underneath, healing will leave a permanent scar.

The skin accurately reflects what is happening elsewhere in the body, and often gives the first indication of an impending illness: the flushed face and sweating of fever; the cold, clammy skin, often with a touch of blueness, of shock; the yellow discolouration of jaundice and the typical rashes of the various infectious fevers. Remember that the common skin diseases listed below are descriptive only. If your child has a persisting or progressive skin rash, it is always wise to consult your doctor to obtain an accurate diagnosis so that the correct treatment can be given.

Skin problems of infancy

Many new babies, particularly those with fine, pale skin, show a bluish mottling of the skin when undressed. Other babies have a deep reddish purple colour on their fingers and hands in the first few weeks of life. Many babies have salmon red marks on their upper eyelids, on the centre of the forehead and at the nape of the neck. These are of no significance and will all disappear completely within the first few months of life.

There are a variety of minor skin rashes that commonly appear in the first few months. They do no harm whatsoever to baby but they naturally concern parents. The most common of these are fine white pearl-like pimples on the face and forehead; small red spots on the cheeks and neck; and little white blisters or loose skin in the centre of the upper or lower lips, produced from vigorous sucking. Some infants, particularly if the skin tends to be a little on the dry side, get rough red patches on the cheeks or forehead that come and go. These things need no treatment and will all clear up completely in a few months.

Prickly heat rash

A baby has very sensitive skin and in hot weather clusters of small pink pimples surrounded by pink blotches sometimes appear on the neck and the upper part of the chest and back. Putting the baby in light clothes to reduce sweating in hot weather will help. Make sure that baby's neck and areas such as the armpits and groin are carefully dried after a bath and apply dusting powder to absorb any additional moisture.

Cradle cap

This is quite common in early infancy and is due to the accumulation of oily secretions from the scalp. It's best managed by daily washing with soap and water followed by the application of baby oil. It rarely persists beyond the first few months of life.

The skin accurately reflects what is happening elsewhere in the body
▼▼▼

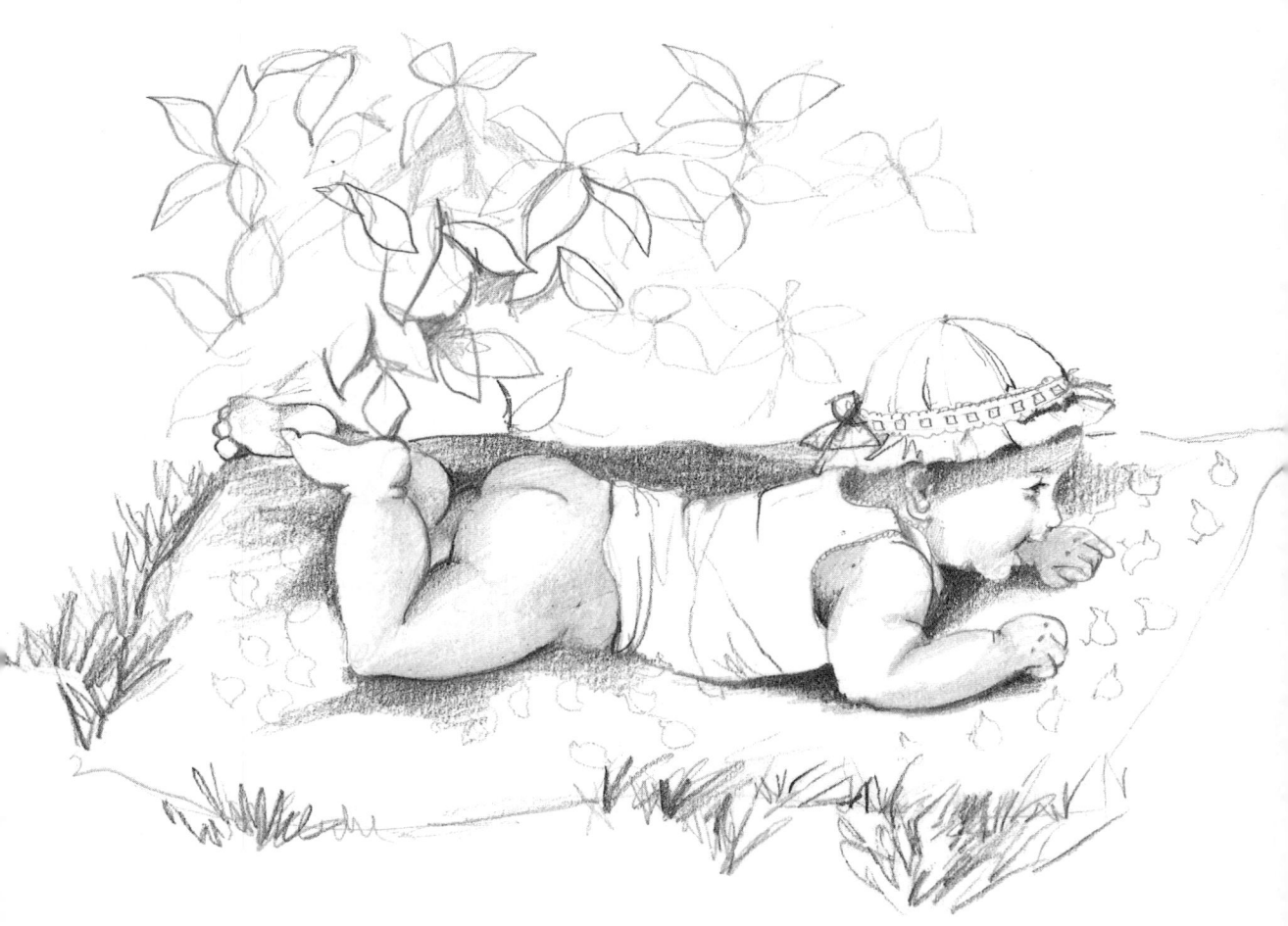

Nappy rash

Almost all babies get some irritation in the nappy area from time to time. It is caused by the irritation from urine and soft motions coming into contact with the baby's tender skin. Most cases will promptly respond to the following simple measures.

- Change wet or dirty nappies promptly. Harmless organisms which live on the skin react with urine to produce ammonia which irritates the skin. The sooner wet nappies are changed, the less time there will be for ammonia to irritate your baby's delicate skin.
- Use only a mild, non-irritating baby soap and be sure to wipe off all soap with water when baby is washed.
- Avoid plastic pants as much as possible. Expose baby without a nappy for 'sun kicks' several times a day. Exposing a nappy rash to the air is the quickest method of getting rid of it.
- If you are using cloth nappies, use a non-irritating soap or detergent and give the nappies a final soak in nappy rinse. Use a soft, lint liner inside the nappy.
- Apply zinc ointment or baby cream to any red areas until they settle.

Thrush

This is a mild fungus infection which occurs in the mouth. It

92   Your Child

looks as if patches of milk are stuck to the tongue, inside the cheeks, or on the roof of the mouth. Thrush can make baby's mouth sore, so that feeding may be less enjoyable. It can easily be treated with drops prescribed by your doctor.

Babies with thrush in the mouth often have it in the nappy area as well. It looks like a nappy rash but one of the main differences is that the rash extends right into the skin creases, areas which are not involved with ordinary nappy rash because they are not in direct contact with urine.

Eczema

In infants, the affected skin feels rough and is pink to red in colour. The rash is patchy and commonly occurs on the cheeks, around the mouth, behind the ears and as the child becomes older it appears in the creases of the elbows, groin, neck and behind the knees. It may be made worse by an external irritant such as wool or the perfume in soap. The rash is very uncomfortable, causing baby to scratch and rub the affected areas.

It's important to seek medical attention as education about avoiding irritants, the use of skin moisteners and creams which counteract the inflammation can bring it under control. Although it improves with time, treatment may be needed for the first few years of life.

SKIN PROBLEMS IN OLDER CHILDREN

Impetigo

Impetigo produces reddish spots, commonly on the face and around the mouth. They produce a clear discharge which rapidly dries to form a honey-coloured crust. The spots spread readily if neglected, and are contagious to other children. It's wise to consult your doctor promptly about impetigo as an oral antibiotic will be needed.

Boils

A boil is due to infection spreading down a hair follicle and causing an abscess. The infection may sometimes spread out below the surface of the skin causing a red, painful, swollen and tender area. Small boils will respond to hot bathing and the application of an antibiotic ointment. However, if the infection seems to be spreading, you should seek medical attention.

Acne

At puberty, the wax glands in the skin become more active, particularly on the face, neck and back. Sometimes, the waxy secretion blocks the outlet of glands which then swell up and become infected. This produces the pimply appearance which is so distressing to many adolescents. With maturity, the condition subsides and completely disappears. When the

Thrush can make baby's mouth sore, so that feeding may be less enjoyable
▼▼▼

pimples become infected and discharge this can result in permanent scarring. The following simple measures will help to keep most cases of acne under control.

- Wash the face and neck several times a day with mild soap and water. Use of an antiseptic soap is helpful in controlling secondary infection.
- Avoid squeezing or scratching the pustules. This only makes them worse.
- Avoid the use of any oily or greasy cosmetic preparations on the face or neck.

If the acne does not respond to these simple measures, your doctor may prescribe a course of tetracycline antibiotic.

Birthmarks
There are several varieties of birthmarks. Some are present when the baby is born, others develop in the first few weeks of life. One of the most common is a red mark on the eyelids and centre of the forehead above the nose. A similar mark may be found at the back of the neck. These marks usually fade within a few months. They are harmless and need no treatment.

The 'strawberry' mark is a raised, red lump. These birthmarks often grow larger for a short time but most of them eventually fade and disappear, usually between the ages of four and five years. The first sign that the mark is going to disappear is when it goes pale at the centre and becomes flatter. Bleeding is not a serious problem and can always be stopped by light pressure. The best cosmetic result is obtained by leaving these marks to fade spontaneously, as surgery will leave a permanent scar.

The birthmark known as the 'port wine stain' is red to purple in colour. It may be flat or slightly raised. These marks remain for life. The best treatment usually is cosmetic, and many cosmetic firms now have experts who will advise parents on the best form of make-up to use to cover the mark. In some cases laser treatment will help.

Moles are brownish-black spots in the skin which are caused by an excess of pigment. In most cases they are quite harmless. However, should a mole change in any way, either by growing larger, becoming darker or more prominent, changing in colour or shape, or bleeding, medical attention should be sought without delay.

Ringworm
This is a fungus infection that may occur either on the scalp or on the body. There is a central pale area surrounded by an irregular ring of reddish skin. The fungus may be caught from dogs, cats or from other affected children. It can be controlled by an appropriate ointment and occasionally by special antibiotics.

> *Should a mole change in any way, medical attention should be sought without delay* ▼▼▼

Warts

Warts are caused by a virus growing in the skin. They most frequently grow on the hands or legs and may be single or multiple. After a variable time, they will disappear spontaneously, which explains why some of the folklore type of wart remedies sometimes seem to work.

If they are unsightly or cause embarrassment, they can be removed by the regular application of a caustic ointment, or can, if necessary, be removed surgically by a doctor.

Bites and stings

Most insect bites are just irritating (mosquitoes and sand-flies) or painful (bees and bull ants). However, some children will develop hives (allergic reactions in the skin) from insect bites. The bites then become inflamed and are very itchy. Usually a soothing lotion such as calamine lotion, and occasionally a mild sedative to prevent scratching at night, are all that is needed.

The most worrying bites are from spiders and snakes. Fortunately these bites are rare. In Australia the red-back and funnel-web spiders are poisonous. Their bites are extremely painful. If you think your child has been bitten by one of these spiders, telephone a children's hospital or poisons information centre for immediate first aid advice and then seek prompt medical treatment.

Most snakes are not poisonous but as even experts may have difficulty identifying snakes, all snake bites should be taken seriously. Fortunately snakes are usually afraid of humans and get out of their way.

Tick bites occur most commonly in the spring and summer when children have been playing in bushland which harbours the insect. If the tick remains unnoticed for several days, it can make the child feel unwell, although tick paralysis, more common in dogs, is rare in humans. Once the tick has been located, it's best killed by applying cotton wool soaked in methylated spirits or kerosene, following which the insect can be carefully extracted with a pair of tweezers.

BONES AND JOINTS

GROWING PAINS

Many school-age children suffer from 'growing pains'. These are not associated with any serious disease. They are typically felt in the mid-portion of the upper and lower legs, but can also sometimes occur in the shoulder and arms. There are no signs of serious joint or limb inflammation. In other words, there is no tenderness, redness, warmth, swelling or limitation of movement of joints or muscles.

After a variable time, warts will disappear spontaneously
▼▼▼

The sick child

These pains are more common in girls than boys, and usually occur between six and twelve years of age. They more commonly occur in the night and the child may wake and cry out with pain.

The cause of the condition is unknown. Many theories have been put forward but none is satisfactory. The term 'growing pains' is not a very accurate one, as the pain is unlikely to be related to growth, but it's the term most commonly used.

The pains usually only last for a short time and often respond to massage and heat. There is no need to limit activity. Occasionally paracetamol may be needed.

Arthritis

Arthritis means inflammation in a joint. The most common form of arthritis in children is a temporary inflammation which follows some viral infections and this type of arthritis always recovers completely. Other types of arthritis can be caused by bacterial infections, which produce a more serious form of arthritis, needing prompt treatment. Occasionally arthritis can be chronic in children, a condition known as JCA, or juvenile chronic arthritis. Because such a wide variety of conditions can cause painful joints in children, it's always wise to have the condition thoroughly checked by a doctor to find the underlying problem.

Club foot (talipes)

There are a number of minor deformities of the foot which may be present at birth. Some require no treatment and others, like overriding toes and inturning of the forefoot, are very simple to correct. However, there is one form of club foot in which one or both feet are twisted severely inwards and backwards and cannot be straightened. This is a very obvious deformity and requires early specialised orthopaedic treatment to straighten the foot. Often this can be done by manipulation and splinting, but in some cases, an operation will be necessary.

Knock-knees and bow legs

Minor degrees of bow legs and knock-knees are so common as to be almost within the normal range. Many children around the age of one year appear to have bow legs because of the prominent fatty tissue on the outer side of their legs and because the thick nappy between their legs affects their posture when walking. It nearly always corrects itself by two years. Other children, when they get their growth spurt, around three years of age, show a degree of knock-knee, often associated with flat feet. This tends to improve spontaneously as the child grows. There is little place for the use of

Minor degrees of bow legs and knock-knees are so common as to be almost normal
▼▼▼

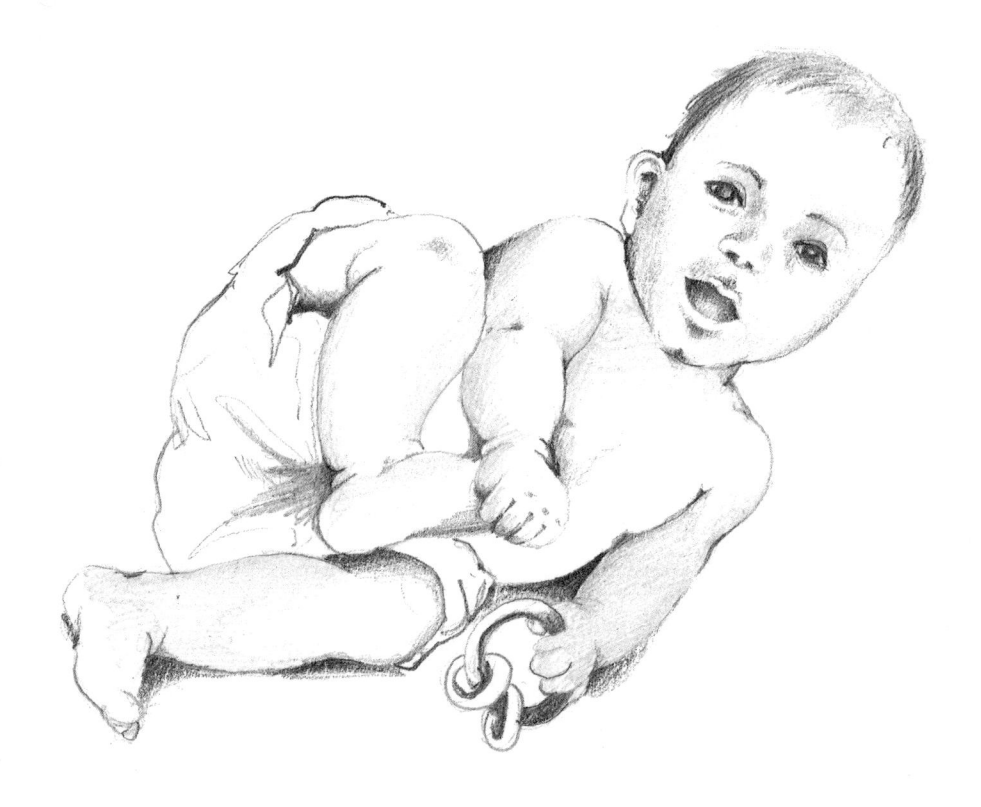

special shoes, or for build-ups on one side of the sole. These conditions are rarely severe enough to require braces or operative treatment and these should never be considered without the advice of an orthopaedic specialist.

Flat feet

All infants have rather fat feet which may look as if they are flat because the fat obscures the arch of the foot. However, the arch can be seen more clearly when the child stands on tiptoes. Other children have fairly loose ligaments in their feet and so do not have an obvious arch.

As they become older the ligaments become firmer and the foot develops its normal arch. Only in rare cases is treatment necessary for flat feet.

Congenital dislocation of the hip

All newborn babies should be checked for this common, potentially crippling condition. If it is found in the first few weeks of life and treated appropriately,

Congenital hip dislocation, if found in the first few weeks of life and treated, does not usually require surgery
▼▼▼

it can usually be completely corrected without the need for surgery. Treatment may require the use of a special brace or sometimes a plaster cast for several months but after this is removed the baby will be able to move normally. The condition now rarely goes undetected so that surgery can usually be avoided by early treatment. In some babies, your doctor may feel that the hip is a little unstable but not actually dislocated. In these cases the baby may need to be nursed in double nappies, thus keeping the legs spread out more than normally or a special harness may need to be worn for a short time. The baby's hips should then be reassessed fairly frequently.

Unstable hips promptly improve during the first month or so of life and are not as serious as a congenital dislocated hip.

SCOLIOSIS

This is a curvature of the spine which usually occurs after the child has commenced the school years, often just around the time of rapid growth at puberty. It is more common in girls. Early detection and treatment are important and scoliosis screening programs are now carried out in the junior years at high schools.

COMMON INFECTIOUS DISEASES

Most of the infectious diseases start with fever. If this is high, it should be reduced by sponging the child with lukewarm water and giving paracetamol in appropriate dosage. Fluids should also be given freely, particularly in hot weather. If your child is vomiting with the fever, give small amounts of fluid at frequent intervals rather than too much at once. Don't worry if your child doesn't want to eat when ill and feverish. The appetite will return to normal once the illness has passed.

All of the common infectious diseases have an incubation period. Towards the end of this incubation period the child becomes vaguely unwell and irritable before the characteristic signs appear. This is the time when the disease is most highly infectious and when other children in the household are most likely to catch it.

It's wise to keep other members of the household away from the infected child unless they have already suffered from that particular disease. This will certainly reduce the risk of them catching it. If other children have been immunised against that particular infectious disease, they will be much less likely to catch it or, if they do so, it will be in a much milder form.

Measles

This has an incubation period of about fourteen days and is most infectious for two or three days before the rash appears. About a week before this, your child may develop a cough, often with red, irritable eyes and fever. After this, the typical rash appears. It is red and blotchy and often appears first on the face and behind the ears. Once the rash appears, the temperature usually subsides within two or three days, and the rash itself rarely lasts for more than four or five days. The main danger of measles is the development of complications such as middle ear infection, bronchitis, pneumonia and occasionally encephalitis. For this reason it is wise for a doctor to see your child to confirm that all is going well.

Because measles is commonly associated with complications, it is very important to have your child immunised against it (see Chapter 4, Immunisation).

Rubella (German measles)

This is a much milder disease than measles. It has an incubation period of two to three weeks but the preliminary symptoms are relatively insignificant. The rash is like that of measles but it only lasts for one or two days. There is usually only a mild fever and no associated cough or sore eyes. One of the distinguishing features is the presence of swollen, tender glands at the back of the neck and behind the ears.

Although rubella is a mild infection, it poses an important risk during pregnancy when it can cause serious damage to the unborn baby. This is why all children should have rubella immunisation at twelve months of age with an extra immunisation given to all girls in their last year of primary school or first year of high school (see Chapter 4, Immunisation).

Mumps

Mumps has an incubation period of two to three weeks. With younger children, the first thing noticed is a swelling just below and in front of the ear. Usually the swelling starts on one side first but within a day or so both sides are usually swollen. Older children sometimes complain of pain when swallowing for a day or so before the swelling appears. They may be generally 'off colour' and there is often a mild fever. The whole illness usually lasts no more than a week. The most common complication is inflammation of the testicles. This is more likely to occur in older children. Less frequently severe abdominal pain and vomiting can result from inflammation of the

Measles rash is red and blotchy and often appears first on the face and behind the ears
▼▼▼

pancreas, and some children may develop encephalitis (inflammation of the brain) which fortunately usually recovers completely. Immunisation at twelve months will protect your child from mumps (see Chapter 4, Immunisation).

Whooping cough

Unlike measles, mumps and rubella, which are caused by viruses, whooping cough is a bacterial disease. This means that antibiotics can have some effect. Although antibiotics do little to affect the course of the illness in a particular child, they do help to stop the condition spreading to other children and family members. The most serious side-effects of whooping cough are on children under the age of twelve months. The incubation period is about two weeks and the infection starts with a mild cough which lasts for a week or so before the cough starts to occur in long, severe bouts, associated with a whoop at the end of the spasm of coughing. In very young children with whooping cough, there may not be a whoop. During a paroxysm of coughing the child may go blue until finally air is drawn into the lungs with a crowing sound, which produces a typical whoop. A bout of coughing is frequently followed by vomiting. Children who have been immunised may sometimes still get whooping cough but usually in a much milder form. The main dangers of the disease are exhaustion from the constant coughing or the development of pneumonia.

Chicken pox

This is also caused by a virus and the incubation period is about two weeks. Symptoms are usually slight, particularly in young children. There may be a little fever at the beginning and older children sometimes feel generally sick and have a headache for a day or so before the spots appear. The rash is very characteristic. It consists of a red patch in the centre of which is a tiny yellowish watery blister which breaks and dries into a scab. New spots continue to appear for four or five days. The rash is itchy and it is difficult to stop the child scratching which may lead to infection and occasionally scarring. A daily bath with oatmeal in the water and the application of a soothing lotion is helpful both in relieving the itching and in preventing secondary infection. Chicken pox is highly contagious so there is a very good chance that other children in the family will catch it and develop the rash at the end of the incubation period. Once there are no new spots appearing, and all the other spots have developed scabs, the child is no longer infectious.

Chicken pox is highly contagious so there is a very good chance that other children in the family will catch it
▼▼▼

Roseola

This viral infection is most common under the age of three. It starts off with high fever for several days. The child feels generally well despite the high temperature. The main problem is that this high temperature may trigger a febrile convulsion in susceptible children. After several days of fever, a rash appears, mainly on the trunk, and the temperature falls at this time. It's basically a mild disease although it may be difficult for the doctor to make a diagnosis during the period of high temperature before the rash appears.

Chest problems

Bronchitis and pneumonia

Bronchitis is an inflammation of the upper airways, usually caused by a virus. It may start off with a dry cough which becomes loose and rattling after a few days and there may be a fever.

The diagnosis of bronchitis is not made as often as it used to be in the past. This is because doctors now realise that the child who has repeated episodes of coughing, associated with shortness of breath most likely is having episodes of asthma. What doctors a generation ago used to call 'wheezy bronchitis' was probably really asthma. Sometimes in bronchitis the infection spreads from the bronchial tubes to cause small patches of inflammation throughout both lungs. This is called broncho-pneumonia. The other form of pneumonia occurs when the virus or bacterial infection is confined to one particular lobe of the lung. This is called lobar pneumonia.

The child with pneumonia is obviously much sicker than she would be with an ordinary cold or bronchitis. There is usually a high fever, and the breathing is rapid and somewhat laboured. There may be a complaint of pain in one part of the chest.

Pneumonia in children is confirmed by an X-ray of the chest and may need to be treated in hospital, with antibiotics given intravenously. Subsequent X-rays may be needed to make sure that the lungs return completely to normal. Once the infection has been brought under control, the material plugging up the bronchial tubes and lungs will loosen and be coughed up. Physiotherapy may help your child get rid of these secretions.

Asthma

Asthma is one of the most common childhood conditions. Up to 20 per cent of children may suffer from it at some time. Asthma, hay fever, and eczema sometimes go together and there are often other family members who have one of these conditions.

Pneumonia in children is confirmed by an X-ray of the chest and may need to be treated in hospital
▼▼▼

Food allergy is not a common cause of asthma
▼▼▼

The most obvious symptom of asthma is wheezing although in some children the main feature may be a night-time cough. The wheezing of asthma is caused by a spasm of the muscles in the small air passages. This is usually accompanied by swelling and the production of mucous in those air passages, which further aggravates the child's difficulty in getting air in and out of the lungs easily.

An episode of asthma is usually triggered by an upper respiratory tract infection or by a sudden change in air temperature. Allergies also play a part in asthma, the most common cause being house dust, something which is hard to avoid. Occasionally emotional upset can trigger an attack. Food allergy is not a common cause of asthma.

If your child has asthma, it's important you discuss this with your doctor so that you can have a thorough understanding of the condition. We know that the more parents and children understand how to interpret and treat the asthma symptoms, the better the asthma is managed. Your doctor should give you a written asthma management plan explaining what sort of treatment to take, when to start taking it and how long to take it. Drug treatment of asthma is of two main types, those which prevent asthma and those which relieve it. Preventive drugs have to be taken on a regular basis, even when the child is well, if they are to be effective. They work by reducing the amount of inflammation in the airways and making the airways less sensitive to some of the things which trigger asthma.

Drugs which relieve asthma are called bronchodilators because they open up the airways to make breathing easier. Children who have only an occasional episode of asthma may only need to take a bronchodilator when they have symptoms whereas children who have more frequent attacks may need regular preventive treatment.

CYSTIC FIBROSIS

This is a serious, inherited disease which affects about one in 2500 children. Numerous body glands are affected. Insufficient digestive juices are secreted by the pancreas and this causes the child to pass frequently bulky stools which smell offensive. The glands supplying the bronchial tubes are also affected so that lung infections occur much more readily and frequently. The sweat glands excrete too much salt and this can be recognised by a 'sweat test' which is useful in making the diagnosis. The child can be given enzyme preparations to make good the deficiency in the digestive juices.

The greatest danger to the child comes from the repeated chest infections which cause permanent lung damage. Treatment involves regular physiotherapy and courses of antibiotics. Because cystic fibrosis is such a complex condition, it is best looked after under the supervision of a special cystic fibrosis clinic; these are conducted at children's hospitals. Since the condition is likely to occur in subsequent pregnancies, families where children have cystic fibrosis need advice about future pregnancies and access to specialist services which are able to make the diagnosis early in pregnancy.

Intestinal problems

Stomach aches

While many diseases cause pain in the abdomen, most complaints of stomach pain in children are not due to disease but are the body's way of expressing some sort of emotional stress in the child, just as headache is in an adult. However, as abdominal pain can sometimes indicate something more serious, a decision has to be made about when to take your child to the doctor. The presence of other symptoms such as vomiting, fever, diarrhoea and frequent passing of urine will mean that a doctor's help is needed.

If, after seeing your doctor, the pain is thought to be due to emotional stress, it's important to understand that your child is not putting it on. As far as the child is concerned the pain is real. Sometimes, you may find the cause readily, such as the child being upset over some family problems or because of difficulties at school. However, at other times, the cause is not found so easily and professional help may be needed if the pains persist or disrupt the child's life. While trying to understand what may be troubling your child and accepting that the pain is real, it's also important not to allow the child to benefit from the pain, such as by missing school, as this may reinforce the symptoms.

Constipation

Constipation is the infrequent passage of abnormally hard motions. It may be quite normal for some children to go two or even three days between bowel actions. This is particularly so with breast-fed babies, but constipation should only be considered to be present if the motions are very hard. Constipation itself doesn't have any serious effects although sometimes it may cause slight bleeding by tearing the delicate skin just inside the anus.

In babies, infrequent bowel motions rarely need treatment, particularly in breast-fed babies. A little extra orange juice or some

If the pain is due to emotional stress, it's important to understand that your child is not putting it on
▼▼▼

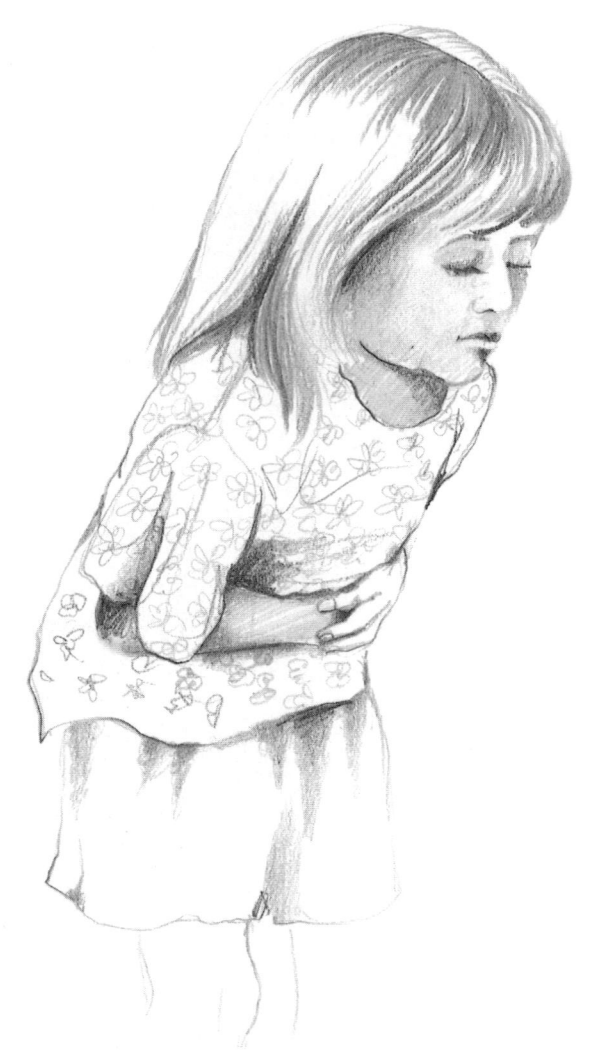

prune juice may prove effective.

In the older child, the most common cause of constipation is a diet lacking sufficient bulk. This can be remedied by giving a cereal containing bran each day. Fruit and vegetables also help.

It should be realised that constipation is sometimes an indication of emotional upset. Little children soon become aware of the fact if parents place too much stress on bowel actions, and they tend to use this as a means of achieving notice. The more importance that is placed on it, the less the child may tend to follow her natural rhythm. Just as some children use mealtime battles as a means of asserting their growing independence, others make use of 'the battle of the bowels'.

If a child retains stools for long enough, some brown liquid material will escape around the hardened collection of stool in the bowel, soiling the underpants. Soiling in older children is a sign of long-standing constipation and should be treated by a doctor.

Vomiting

Persistent vomiting in a small baby can be due to many causes — infection, in association with diarrhoea in gastroenteritis or due to some more serious surgical problem. All babies vomit or posset a little from time to time and this is often called reflux. If vomiting persists and is copious then your doctor should be consulted promptly. It is important to realise that vomiting is not due to breast-feeding or to an unsuitable brand of milk, and there is nothing to be gained in changing from one to another. If baby is gaining weight satisfactorily, the vomiting is not likely to be serious. However, if it is persistent you should consult your doctor without delay.

Diarrhoea and vomiting — gastroenteritis

A small infant's bowels are easily upset and diarrhoea, consisting of frequent greenish motions, can occur with a cold or when certain fruits or vegetables are introduced into the diet for the first time. However, such attacks are quite mild and usually settle down within a day or so. Baby is not upset during such an attack although the loose motions may temporarily irritate the skin around the anus.

Gastroenteritis is more severe than this. There is usually vomiting as well as watery greenish diarrhoea and the motions may contain mucus or blood. There is often a fever. Baby looks sick and is listless, with sunken eyes and dry skin and passes less urine than normal.

If the vomiting and diarrhoea are severe, there is considerable fluid loss and the baby rapidly becomes dehydrated. Under such circumstances, it will usually be advisable to admit the child to hospital for fluid replacement.

Although there are bacteria that cause specific types of gastroenteritis, most cases are due to a viral infection and therefore they don't respond to antibiotics. Gastroenteritis is uncommon while babies are being breast fed.

If your baby has more than a transient attack of diarrhoea it's wise to consult you doctor without delay or to take baby to a children's hospital for treatment. If the condition is not severe enough to require admission to hospital, the most important part of treatment is the replacement of the fluid that is being lost. To reduce the chance of vomiting, it's better to give small drinks frequently rather than large quantities. If you are breast-feeding, continue to do so. Solutions containing some of the chemicals lost with gastroenteritis, such as Gastrolyte, can be obtained in pharmacies and can be given by mouth to help replace the fluid loss. Juices or soft drinks may actually increase diarrhoea in infants and should not be given in

There are no medications that are safe or effective for gastroenteritis in children
▼▼▼

full strength. They can be used if diluted with one part of juice to three parts of water. There are no medications that are safe or effective for gastroenteritis in children. The mainstay of treatment is fluid replacement.

Gastroenteritis is less of a problem in older children and can usually be easily looked after at home, but because infants can become dehydrated very quickly, they need to be assessed and treated under medical supervision.

Appendicitis

Whenever your child complains of abdominal pain, it's natural to worry in case this might be due to appendicitis. Appendicitis is uncommon under the age of two and difficult to diagnose under the age of four years. The signs that should alert you to the possibility of appendicitis, whenever your child complains of abdominal pain, are loss of appetite, particularly if this is associated with nausea or vomiting, and any sudden alteration in bowel habit — constipation or diarrhoea. The pain in appendicitis usually starts above or around the navel, and only later in the attack does it move to the right lower side of the abdomen. At this stage it becomes associated with tenderness in that area. Although most abdominal pain in children is not of a serious nature, you should be concerned if it persists or recurs, or if any of the above signs are present. You should also be concerned if it occurs at night, particularly if it wakes your child from sleep. If in any doubt as to the pain's origin, consult your doctor.

Worms

Threadworms are the common variety. They cause irritation around the anus and sometimes redness and vaginal discharge in little girls. The irritation may make the child restless at night, when the worms tend to come out between the buttocks. If you inspect the area with a torch at this time, you may see the worms, which look like fine white threads about 1 cm long.

Less commonly, children suffer from roundworms which look very much like small earthworms. They usually don't cause any symptoms but may be noticed in the motions. In either case, your doctor can prescribe treatment which will promptly eradicate the worms. It is usually wise to treat all children in the family at the same time since they are often all affected. In most instances, worms do not cause any symptoms unless the child has a great number of them.

The pain in appendicitis usually starts above or around the navel
▼▼▼

Kidney and bladder problems

Infections of the bladder and kidneys

Urine is produced by the kidneys and passed into the bladder where it's stored until it's convenient to pass it. When urine becomes infected, the bladder is irritated and this causes a frequent desire to pass urine, often only in small amounts. Passing urine often causes a stinging or burning sensation. Your child may be feverish and complain of pain in the lower abdomen over the bladder.

Infants may have bladder or kidney infections with very few symptoms. Recurrent fever for no obvious reason and failure to grow normally may be the only signs.

If the kidneys as well as the bladder are infected, the child is usually sicker and sometimes complains of backache. Infection of the kidney, if it's allowed to continue unchecked, can produce permanent damage to the kidney. It's therefore important that kidney infection is detected early in order to prevent serious and progressive damage to the kidneys.

Kidney and bladder infections are more common in girls than in boys, and persisting or recurrent infections are sometimes associated with some congenital abnormality in the urine collecting system or the kidneys.

Infection of the urine can only be diagnosed by growing bacteria from a properly collected specimen. It's not possible to tell merely by looking at the urine whether it is infected. A normal child may have cloudy urine but if this is persistent, and particularly if the smell of the urine is offensive, it's wise to consult your doctor.

Children who have a urine infection which is proven by growing the bacteria should have their bladder and kidneys evaluated, usually by ultrasound and X-rays to make sure that there is no underlying problem in the urinary tract which may need more extensive treatment and regular medical supervision.

Nephritis

This is the word used to describe a group of disorders which affect the filtering system in the kidneys. Most children with nephritis recover completely. Nephritis is most commonly seen following a throat or skin infection with the streptococcus bacteria. Streptococcal infections are common and usually are not associated with nephritis. Occasionally, however, one or two weeks after the infection, the child is noticed to have a puffy face and the amount of urine passed is reduced and smoky in colour. This is due to the presence of blood in the urine which, after

Kidney and bladder infections are more common in girls than in boys
▼▼▼

being in the bladder, changes from red to a dark brown colour. The child may also develop headache, fever and vomiting.

The illness usually lasts two to three weeks and during this time, fluid and diet restrictions will be necessary. In most cases, the attack is relatively mild and your child can be treated at home providing a close check is kept on the amount of urine passed, the body weight and the blood pressure.

If the illness is more severe or prolonged it will be necessary for your child to be admitted to hospital where further tests will be carried out. Although some forms of nephritis occasionally produce permanent kidney damage, the majority of cases recover completely.

Genital Disorders

Vaginal discharge

A small amount of clear or white mucus is normally produced by the young girl's vagina. If it's enough to produce soiling of the underwear, it's usually due to a minor infection which will clear up spontaneously in a short time. However, if the discharge is thick, very smelly, copious or blood-stained, you should seek advice from your doctor without delay. Beads, plastic toys and similar objects are sometimes placed in the natural body cavities, including the vagina, by curious children. This will always cause a discharge. Many young children go through a phase of exploring their own bodies and this not infrequently includes poking objects into the nose, ears, anus or vagina.

Poor hygiene, or local irritation sometimes caused by threadworms can also contribute to a discharge from the vagina. One of the most common causes of local irritation is the perfume found in some soaps and bubble baths which irritates this sensitive area. Avoiding bubble baths or changing to a mild, non-perfumed soap may solve the problem.

Occasionally a discharge can result from gonorrhoea, as a result of sexual contact. This is something you may not want to think about, and sometimes children are too frightened to discuss these experiences even with their parents. This is an area where a paediatrician can be of great help.

Circumcision

Circumcision is the operation of removing most of the foreskin. Occasionally it is necessary to perform this operation to treat recurrent infection under the foreskin or excessive narrowing of the opening in the foreskin. Many parents don't realise that the opening of the foreskin is

As your little boy gets bigger, the opening in the foreskin enlarges naturally
▼▼▼

usually too small to allow it to be drawn back over the head of the penis and that it's normally slightly stuck on to the end of the penis for the first few years of life. As your little boy gets bigger, the opening in the foreskin enlarges naturally and the skin separates from the end of the penis so that it can be drawn back with ease. Before this is possible, the only care necessary is to wash the penis normally in the bath without attempting to draw the foreskin back.

Apart from religious reasons, most boys do not need circumcision. It's not necessary for proper cleanliness. All operations carry some risk and circumcision is no exception. It should not be done unless necessary. The operation carries greater risks in the newborn baby and is best avoided at that time. If for any reason you want your son to be circumcised, it's better to defer it until he is out of nappies.

Hernia and hydrocele

Umbilical hernia, or protrusion of the navel, is very common, occurring in about one in five children. It causes unnecessary concern to many parents. In most cases it undergoes spontaneous cure, disappearing during the first two or three years of life. It is not associated with any symptoms or complications. If it is still obvious at the age of three years, it can be corrected by a simple operation.

A hernia in the groin (inguinal hernia) on the other hand, will not get better by itself. Sometimes, a loop of bowel can be caught up in the hernia and become obstructed and this may require urgent operation. An inguinal hernia is noticed as a swelling in the groin which may extend down into the scrotum. Sometimes it is present at birth, in other cases it may not appear until later in childhood. If you notice any swelling in the groin of your child, consult your doctor. A simple operation can prevent worrying complications from occurring. This should be done as soon as convenient after the hernia is discovered.

A hydrocele is a sack of fluid surrounding the testis. It's not uncommon in small infants and in such cases usually disappears spontaneously by the age of six months. When it occurs in older children, or if it does not disappear spontaneously in a small infant, a simple operation can correct the condition. Sometimes it's associated with an inguinal hernia which can be dealt with at the same time.

Undescended testis

The testis actually develops inside the abdomen and does not come to lie in its final position in the scrotum until shortly before birth. In many small boys, the testes will be temporarily pulled up into

Umbilical hernia is very common and usually disappears spontaneously during the first two or three years of life
▼▼▼

the groin by a band of muscle along the spermatic cord. This is quite normal. If you have any doubt as to whether the testis is in its correct site, examine your child when he is relaxed in a warm bath. In this situation the testis should be lying in the scrotum.

Any boy over the age of one year in whom both testes are not obviously in the scrotum should be checked by your doctor. After this age the testis will not come down spontaneously. If the testis is not in the scrotum during childhood it's less likely to develop normally. It will still produce male sex hormones so that your child will mature normally, but it's less likely to produce sperm and therefore may not be fertile. If both testes are undescended, this could cause sterility although it will not interfere with the child maturing and having normal sexual activity.

If the testis is undescended it has to be brought down into the scrotum to give it the best chance of developing normally. Surgeons differ about the best time for the operation, with some believing it is best done before two years, but it certainly should be done before five years of age. The procedure is not a major operation but is best done by a surgeon experienced in the procedure and can usually be done as a 'day-stay' operation.

The majority of tumours can be cured by a combination of surgery with chemotherapy or radiotherapy ▼▼▼

MALIGNANT DISEASE

Cancer in childhood is quite different from the types of cancer seen in adult life. One third of the cancers of childhood are leukaemia, one fifth are brain tumours and most of the remainder are tumours growing in or near the kidneys or in the lymph glands. The disease usually starts very insidiously with vague symptoms such as loss of weight, headache and paleness. If your child continues to complain of any of these symptoms, is persistently unwell or develops any unexplained lump or continuing pain, check with your doctor. It should be stressed that malignant disease is very rare in childhood but can be extremely serious. It tends to progress rapidly and spread early. The cause of malignant disease is not known but it's not inherited and cannot be passed on to other children. It's very rare for it to occur more than once in a family.

There have been great advances in the treatment of childhood cancer. The majority of tumours can be cured by a combination of surgery with chemotherapy or radiotherapy. Well over half the children who suffer from acute leukaemia are able to have the condition cured by a combination of powerful drugs and sometimes with bone marrow transplant. However, all of these treatments are prolonged and complex. While these conditions remain very serious and not always amenable to treatment, it is known that the chances of success are best if the treatment is given and supervised by one of the special cancer (oncology) units based at a children's hospital.

CONGENITAL MALFORMATIONS

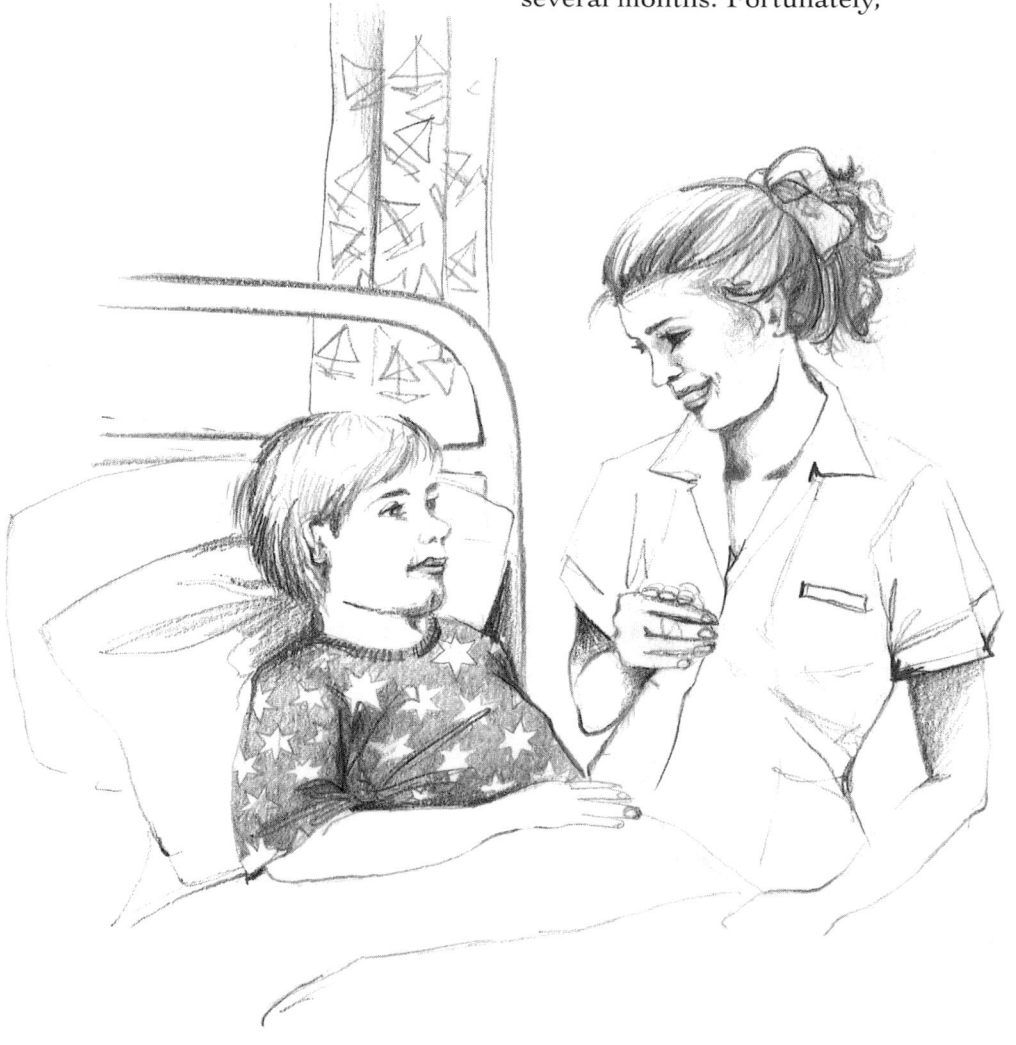

These are defects of formation of the body that are present at birth. About 2 per cent of all babies are born with serious congenital defects sufficient to threaten life, cause handicap or need surgical correction. Most defects are detected soon after birth but some do not become evident for several months. Fortunately, nature spontaneously terminates many pregnancies in which the developing foetus has a serious malformation.

What is the cause of congenital defects? The true story is not yet fully known. Abnormalities of genes and chromosomes cause quite a large proportion. Occasionally some congenital malformations are more common in particular ethnic groups, some are more common in children of older parents and others tend to run in families.

Other potentially hazardous agents are: radiation, including excessive use of X-rays during pregnancy; drugs taken during pregnancy such as thalidomide and quinine; and infections such as rubella.

What is important to understand is that these defects are usually not due to anything the mother may have done, or neglected to do during pregnancy. Major advances are being made in understanding the genetic background which leads to many congenital malformations. Quite a number of these conditions can now be detected early in pregnancy by techniques known as amniocentesis or chorionic villus sampling. This can be particularly valuable if there is a family history of the condition or if a previous child with the condition has been born to the parents. As new knowledge in this area is being gained every week, it's important, if there is a family history of an inherited condition, to seek advice from a genetic counselling service, such as the ones based at children's hospitals.

When a major abnormality is detected after birth, expert paediatric help should be sought immediately. The parents should be told whether the condition can be corrected, any residual handicap the baby will have and whether it is likely to recur in a further pregnancy.

In all such cases, the parents will need considerable support and advice to help them adjust to an unexpected, distressing situation and to keep them fully informed about what is being done for their baby. When the condition is an inherited one, they'll need to be carefully and accurately advised about the chances of recurrence so that they'll be able to decide what they want to do about further pregnancies.

Following are some congenital malformations and diseases seen in the first few months of life.

CONGENITAL HEART DISEASE

This is one of the most common major congenital malformations. Some of these infants are 'blue babies' while in others the colour can be normal. Some babies are born with a hole between two of the chambers of the heart or with severe narrowing between the

Major advances are being made in understanding the genetic background to many congenital malformations
▼▼▼

heart and one of the major blood vessels.

Congenital heart disease, although it may be severe and even life-threatening, may not be obvious at birth. Sometimes, failure to grow, feeding difficulties or breathlessness are the only obvious signs. Whenever congenital heart disease is suspected, a specialist paediatrician should be consulted or, if the baby is seriously ill, the cardiac team at a children's hospital should see the baby promptly. Remarkable advances have taken place and the majority of children, even with complicated forms of congenital heart disease, can be completely cured.

MALFORMATIONS OF THE BOWEL, KIDNEY AND LUNGS

When serious congenital malformations affecting these organs are present, it will be necessary for baby to be transferred to a specialist children's hospital. The safe care of these tiny infants requires the co-ordinated management of a team of specialists. Sometimes the abnormalities are multiple, affecting many different organs in the body and in some of these cases it may not be either possible or advisable to undertake surgery.

All of this is very confusing and distressing for the parents. Their new baby, which was going to bring them so much happiness, is not only sick but if they live in the country may have been suddenly swept away from them, perhaps several hundred kilometres, to a new, strange and perhaps at first overwhelming hospital amongst a strange group of doctors with whom the parents have had no previous association. The important process of bonding that should be going on between mother and her new baby has been seriously disturbed. As soon as it can be arranged, mother and, if possible, father, should travel to the children's hospital to be with their baby. Arrangements can always be made under these circumstances for mother, and often father too, to have accommodation at the hospital to be close to the baby. The specialist in charge of the baby's problem, will make sure that the parents are kept fully informed, and as soon as baby's medical condition allows, the parents can participate in the care of their new baby. In this way these important early relationships will be disturbed as little as possible.

CLEFT LIP AND CLEFT PALATE

The cleft lip, although the most obvious deformity and therefore the most upsetting to parents, is, in fact, the least serious. It can be repaired before the age of three months and the scar is usually not very obvious. Surgery is only delayed for this length of time to enable the baby to start gaining

Congenital heart disease may not be obvious at birth
▼▼▼

weight and to make the operation safer.

The more serious deformity is the cleft palate. This is a defect in the roof of the mouth. It may interfere with feeding early in life and later on there can be problems with speech development. The best results are usually obtained by repairing the palate between the ages of twelve and eighteen months. This allows the palate time to grow and the result is usually very satisfactory. Most of these babies will feed quite successfully. Any difficulties may be overcome by using a special teat. Arrangements will be made for your child to attend a cleft palate clinic where the services of a number of specialists are available to deal with any associated problems, such as hearing difficulties, speech defects, and any associated dental problems which often accompany the more severe types of cleft palate.

Spina bifida

This serious condition involves the brain, spinal cord and central nervous system, and the bones of the spinal column. In most cases, baby is born with an obvious reddish, raised swelling over the lower part of the spine. This is usually associated with severe weakness of both legs and interference with the function of the bladder and bowel. Control of urinary and bowel activities is likely to be defective.

Unfortunately, the paralysis associated with the condition is likely to be permanent. Sometimes these children die soon after birth. Those likely to survive should be referred to a specialised unit in a children's hospital since their continuing management will be prolonged and complicated. A spina bifida clinic at a children's hospital can help to co-ordinate the work of all the specialists who will be involved in the child's care and can also provide practical support and advice.

Hydrocephalus

Hydrocephalus or 'water on the brain' may be associated with spina bifida or may occur independently. If baby's head appears unduly large or seems to be growing at an excessively rapid rate, expert medical attention should be sought. A variety of investigations will be carried out to find the underlying cause and then surgical correction can usually be done. Early detection of hydrocephalus should enable the condition to be arrested before damage to the developing brain occurs.

Early detection of hydrocephalus should enable it to be arrested before damage to the developing brain occurs
▼▼▼

Some other childhood illnesses

Febrile convulsions

This is a fit or convulsion occurring in response to a high temperature. It occurs most commonly from the age of six months to five years, and rarely after the age of five. About 3 per cent of children are susceptible to febrile convulsions.

The cause for the high fever which irritates the child's brain and causes these convulsions is usually a viral infection such as a cold. Teething does not cause convulsions, nor does constipation. There is often a history of another child in the family or a close relative having been similarly affected. Less than half of all children who have a short febrile convulsion will experience a second one and less than half who experience a second will ever have a third.

Convulsions are frightening and are extremely distressing to the parents. The child who has a high temperature usually stiffens and then twitches, the whole body shakes, the mouth clenches and there may be some blueness around the mouth. Only rarely is the tongue bitten. The duration of this convulsion is usually short — less than five minutes. Afterwards, the child is often drowsy and may sleep. Sometimes the bowels open or urine is passed during the fit.

It's important to stay with the child during the convulsion and not to panic or rush off for help. Protect the child's head and limbs by preventing them from hitting any hard objects during the jerking. Lie the child on the side and keep the airway open by moving the head backwards slightly to extend the neck. There is no need to force the child's mouth open, this is just likely to damage the teeth. Once the fit is over, this is the time to seek help and to contact the doctor or take the child to hospital. As a convulsion and high temperature can sometimes be the first sign of a serious underlying problem, such as meningitis, it's wise to have a careful medical check.

Febrile convulsions only occur in the presence of a high fever, so that it's necessary to reduce the fever, particularly in the age group from six months to three years. Remove clothing, commence sponging with lukewarm water and give paracetamol, to help to lower the temperature. Although these measures are best undertaken before a convulsion occurs, they can also be applied after the child has stopped convulsing, to get the temperature down.

Although febrile convulsions look frightening, they do not cause any brain damage and are not related to epilepsy.

> *Febrile convulsions only occur in the presence of a high fever*
> ▼▼▼

Allergy means an abnormal sensitivity to a particular substance which is normally harmless
▼▼▼

ALLERGIES

Allergy is a word that is frequently misused. Allergy really means an abnormal sensitivity to a particular substance which is normally harmless, so that whenever the allergic child comes into contact with this substance a reaction occurs. This allergic reaction can occur in various parts of the body, such as the skin (hives), the nose and eyes (hay fever), in the lungs (asthma) or in the digestive tract (causing diarrhoea and vomiting). Parents often want to blame a particular food for their child's illness, but usually allergy is not the cause. Allergy tests may sometimes be helpful, but often the parents' own observation can be best. If you notice that your child always has an allergic reaction to a particular food, then it's best to avoid that food.

Much is written about cow's milk allergy, although it's not as common here in Australia as the popular magazines would suggest. Infants sometimes develop rashes or diarrhoea for a variety of reasons and sometimes these are unfairly blamed on the milk, especially if the condition spontaneously clears up at the same time as the milk is changed. True cow's milk allergy does occur in a small number of children. Symptoms almost invariably start during the first two to three months of life and usually begin within a few days after starting cow's milk or cow's milk-based artificial milk mixtures. Vomiting, diarrhoea and poor weight gain are the major features of milk allergy. Some babies may have a skin rash and persistent cough as well. Most children with cow's milk allergy are able to tolerate cow's milk after the age of two years. If you are worried about your child being allergic to cow's milk, consult your doctor. The best way to avoid it is to entirely breast feed the baby for at least the first few months.

FAILURE TO THRIVE

There is considerable variation in the rate at which normal babies gain weight. Although the average baby is around 3.5 kg at birth, a weight of 2.5 kg or 4 kg may still be well within the normal range. Your doctor or clinic sister can judge whether baby is gaining adequately in weight and height by reference to a percentile chart. This shows the range of normal weight and height at different ages. As long as your child is running along a line within the normal range, there's no cause for concern.

Most parents find it helpful to visit the baby health centre at regular intervals so that baby's progress may be measured and they can receive reliable advice about introducing new foods into her diet. You will have an opportunity to ask any questions about her general management.

When you visit the baby health centre, a check will be kept on your baby's height, weight and head growth. If slow weight gain continues for no obvious reason, it's time to seek expert advice from your doctor.

There are many reasons why infants fail to thrive. The first thing to check is that their food intake is adequate. Are they getting enough food of sufficient variety?

If they are not gaining satisfactorily and still appear hungry at the end of a feed, try them with a little more. Persistent vomiting or loose bulky motions may also be a cause of failure to thrive, and indicate the need for medical advice. Sometimes, infants have some hidden congenital malformation of which the parents are unaware and which may not have been obvious in the newborn period. Some forms of congenital heart disease and malformations of the kidneys, lungs, liver and other important organs can be associated with poor weight gain and this may be the only obvious symptom.

Infants also seem to grow better when they get lots of love and attention. As well as needing enough of the right foods to eat, they need plenty of 'emotional nutrition' to help their growth and development.

Meningitis

Within the skull, the brain is surrounded by a sheet of tissue called the meninges. The space between the meninges and the surface of the brain is filled with cerebrospinal fluid (CSF). This layer of fluid between the brain and the surrounding bony skull helps to protect the brain from injury. The fluid also keeps the surface of the brain moist and healthy. The meninges and the CSF extend down through the backbone around the spinal cord.

Meningitis is usually due to a bacterial infection and is a very serious illness. Although most children recover completely with modern treatment, long-term complications can still occur. These can include deafness, learning problems or more permanent effects on brain function.

About half the cases of serious, bacterial meningitis have been due to the haemophilus influenza type B bacteria (HIB). With the availability of HIB immunisation for children, most of these particular cases of meningitis will be able to be prevented. This is another reason why it is so important to have your child immunised (see Chapter 4, Immunisation).

Some cases of meningitis are due to a viral infection and this usually recovers completely.

The disease starts with fever, headache, vomiting, drowsiness and a stiff neck. In small infants,

Infants seem to grow better when they get lots of love and attention
▼▼▼

the early symptoms may be less obvious. A fit or convulsion may occur. Any child with symptoms suggestive of meningitis requires prompt medical attention.

Children who catch meningitis are usually otherwise normal.

Epilepsy

Epilepsy is the name given to repeated convulsions that occur without any obvious cause, such as fever or infection. Rarely epilepsy may be due to a brain tumour or may result from an injury to the brain. In the great majority of cases, however, the cause is unknown. In major (grand mal) epilepsy, there is a generalised convulsion which involves both arms and legs. The child suddenly becomes unconscious and all the muscles are rigid. After a few seconds, generalised jerking commences. At this time, urine may be passed and the bowels may open. The convulsive movements may last for several minutes. The child then relaxes, may wake briefly and then usually falls into a deep sleep lasting several hours.

It's important to ensure that during the fit the child is not injured by bumping against furniture. Never leave the child unattended during an attack. The head should be turned to one side and pulled backwards slightly to keep the airway open. If the convulsive movements persist, the child must be taken promptly to hospital where oxygen will be administered and anticonvulsant drugs given to control the fit. Petit mal epilepsy is one of the minor forms of epilepsy. It is confined to children. In this type of epilepsy, there is no jerking convulsion. The child stops what she is doing and stares vacantly. The attacks usually only last a few seconds after which the child continues whatever she was doing completely unaware of the attack. The frequency of the attacks varies but they may occur several times a day.

There are a variety of other forms of minor epilepsy which are best sorted out by a paediatrician.

The diagnosis of epilepsy is made by a special examination of the brain's electrical activity, an electroencephalogram (EEG), some blood tests and often a brain scan. Children with recurrent attacks of major or minor epilepsy require treatment with anticonvulsant drugs for several years and should be regularly reviewed. This results in control of the convulsions in the great majority of children, who can then lead a normal life.

Diabetes

In this condition, the pancreas is unable to produce enough insulin. Insulin is a hormone which is necessary for the proper utilisation of sugar (glucose) by the body. There is a tendency for

Insulin is a hormone which is necessary for the proper utilisation of sugar by the body
▼▼▼

diabetes to run in families. Although it's more common in older people, about 5 per cent of cases occur before the age of fifteen years.

In children, it usually has a rapid onset and the child may suddenly become ill and drowsy or lapse into a coma. All young diabetics need careful medical supervision and they require insulin, which can only be given by injection. A carefully controlled diet is a very important part of management. Both parents and the child need to understand the disease and what is required to keep the child in good health. Special clinics are available in all children's hospitals to undertake the continuing care of these children.

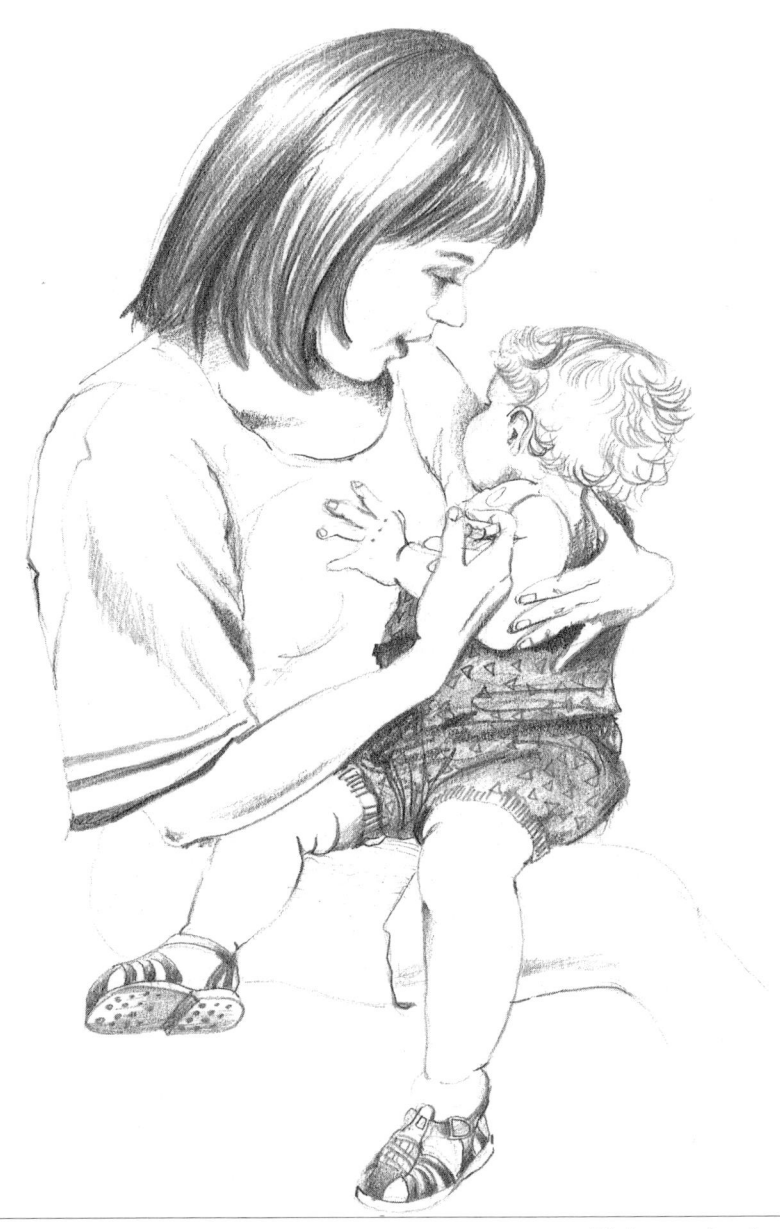

The Sudden Infant Death Syndrome (SIDS)

The Sudden Infant Death Syndrome or cot death causes one to two deaths for every one thousand babies born alive. It can affect babies from two weeks to two years old but the most common age group is one to seven months of age.

What causes sudden infant death? Although the condition has been studied extensively, the cause is unknown. It is certainly not due to suffocation, choking or neglect. The condition has been known for a long time and is not due to drugs or to any new developments. It is not increasing in frequency. It is more apparent now because most of the major causes of death in infants have been overcome.

It can occur in any family, and to the most caring and loving parents. The death is not the fault of the parent, relative, baby-sitter or doctor caring for the child. It can even happen while children are being cared for in hospital. It is not hereditary and is very unlikely to occur again in the same family. It is not catching. Most of these babies are completely healthy beforehand but some may have had a minor illness such as a cold or tummy upset.

Naturally the parents are shocked and shattered by this sudden tragedy. They often feel very guilty because they think they must have missed the signs of some serious illness which should have prompted them to call the doctor. This is not so; and even if the doctor had been called, there would have been no reason to order any treatment since the tragedy could not have been anticipated.

Recent research has shown that the incidence of SIDS can be reduced when babies are breast fed, kept in a smoke-free environment and not allowed to be so wrapped and covered up that they become too hot when asleep. The most important new finding is that the risk is reduced when babies are put to sleep on their side or back rather than on their stomach.

It is important when a tragic event such as SIDS occurs that the parents should be offered expert counselling and support so they can come to understand their confusion and distress. This is best arranged through an understanding family doctor or a specialist paediatrician and the help of the Sudden Infant Death Association.

The death is not the fault of the parent, relative, baby-sitter or doctor caring for the child ▼▼▼

CHAPTER 9

GOING TO HOSPITAL

Going to hospital and having surgery can have disturbing psychological and emotional effects on a child, but today hospitalisation is much less traumatic.

For babies a major factor is separation from Mum and this is one important reason to encourage mothers to spend as much time with their babies as possible and to help in their care. In the first weeks of life, being together helps to develop and preserve the important bond between a mother and her baby, but parents worry much less if at least one of them can be there to see what is happening and to comfort their child.

Toddlers are much more complex. A toddler at home can make his parents understand his wishes. It's much more difficult for him to tell a nurse or other stranger in hospital what he wants. If a parent is with him though, it's still possible for the toddler to communicate and be comforted, especially when he is in pain. Toddlers vary enormously in the extent to which they depend on their mothers and fathers. Whereas some small children are placid, outgoing and amenable, others are apprehensive and get upset when in strange surrounds, particularly when there is no-one familiar around.

Young children may fantasise that being sent to hospital and the pain of surgery are punishment for something they did wrong. School-age children, although they may not admit it, have much the same fears. They have learnt to fear and may think of surgery, and particularly anaesthesia, in terms of dying.

PREPARATION FOR HOSPITAL

Preparation for hospital should start in the doctor's surgery. It is better for both parents to be present and to be told in everyday language what is wrong with their child, what is going to be done and why it's necessary for him to go to hospital. This explanation should include any tests that are necessary before the child is admitted. If an operation is required, this should also be described in simple terms and the parents should know approximately how long the child is likely to be in hospital. School-age children should be included in the explanation. If the reason for admission relates to some serious illness, it may be better to discuss it fully with the parents alone first, particularly if

Parents can play hospital games with their child to help him understand what is going to happen
▼▼▼

the explanation is likely to be distressing to them. But whether the discussion is held with both parents and child simultaneously or if the doctor talks to the child after the parents, a simple factual discussion should be held so that the child knows well in advance what is planned. With toddlers it is better to leave the explanation to the parents, who'll know how much he'll understand. In young children this is best deferred until a day or so before the planned admission. But it's important to stress to the parents that explanation is necessary. The child must not be deceived and must not lose faith in his parents.

The doctor and medical instruments must never be used as a threat to the child — parents have been known to say, 'If you don't behave yourself, the doctor will give you a needle.' Deceptions must never be used — for example, 'I haven't the heart to tell him he's going to hospital, I'll just say we're going for a holiday.' Such practices are foolish. One must never break the trust between a doctor and his little patient, and above all one must never destroy the trust and reliance that exist between parent and child.

Some admissions to hospital are urgent and unexpected. In this situation preparation is not possible and it's best for a parent to be with the child to support him, answer his questions and comfort him.

PREPARATION BY PLAY

Children often show their feelings and fears through play. Parents can play hospital games with their child and his toys to help him understand what is going to happen. For example, games about doctors and nurses could include pretending to give needles and putting on bandages. Colouring books and story books about going to hospital are also useful.

ANSWERING QUESTIONS

A child's questions about going to hospital should be answered simply and accurately and in a way that he can understand. For example, if he asks questions about needles, he should be told that doctors sometimes need to give him medicines in this way or to take a small sample of blood. He should be told it's like a pin prick and that it will only hurt for a moment. Never tell him it won't hurt — it does.

Children will sometimes ask how long they are going to stay in hospital. It's better not to give them an exact date as this can change. It's better to say, if this is true, that they are staying for a few days or that they'll be going home as soon as they're better. If parents are unsure of the answer to their child's questions they should say that they'll ask the nurse or doctor to help answer them. Remember, questions may need to be answered several times, but make sure that your answers are truthful and consistent.

Explaining facts

Children, particularly school-age children, can have confused ideas about an operation or anaesthesia. They find it hard to understand how they can be made to go to sleep and why they won't wake up if somebody touches or hurts them. They should also be told about any special tests they may have. For instance if a child is going to have an X-ray, he can be told that this is like having a picture taken. You should also make it clear that he will not feel well immediately after an operation, that there'll be some discomfort, but that the doctors and nurses will help by giving him medicine to prevent him from having too much pain. Brothers and sisters should also be included in the explanation. They may share the patient's worries and wonder if the same thing is likely to happen to them.

If the doctor doesn't tell you how your child will look when you first see him after surgery in the recovery room, ask him. You need to know if there will be tubes in him and especially if there will be life support devices such as ventilators.

Pre-admission visiting

Children's hospitals welcome visits by parents and children before the child actually comes to hospital. Some children's hospitals run discussion groups for parents to assist them in preparing themselves and their child for hospitalisation. With an apprehensive or dependent child, it's often helpful to visit the hospital and ward shortly before coming to hospital so that you and your child can know and talk about what is going to happen. You can meet the staff and see where the child will eat and sleep and play. This is likely to reduce the child's fears and fantasies about hospital and will help you to understand the hospital. It's nice to know where you're going when you arrive for surgery — it's a time when everyone is tense and worried.

What to take to hospital

It's useful for the child to help pack his own bag, including special toys and other reminders of home. These should be well marked with his name. Many children have a special cuddly or familiar toy which should always go with them, no matter how old or grubby it is. It's very important for them to have this special reminder of home at this time.

It's often helpful to visit the hospital and ward shortly before coming to the hospital
▼▼▼

Going to hospital

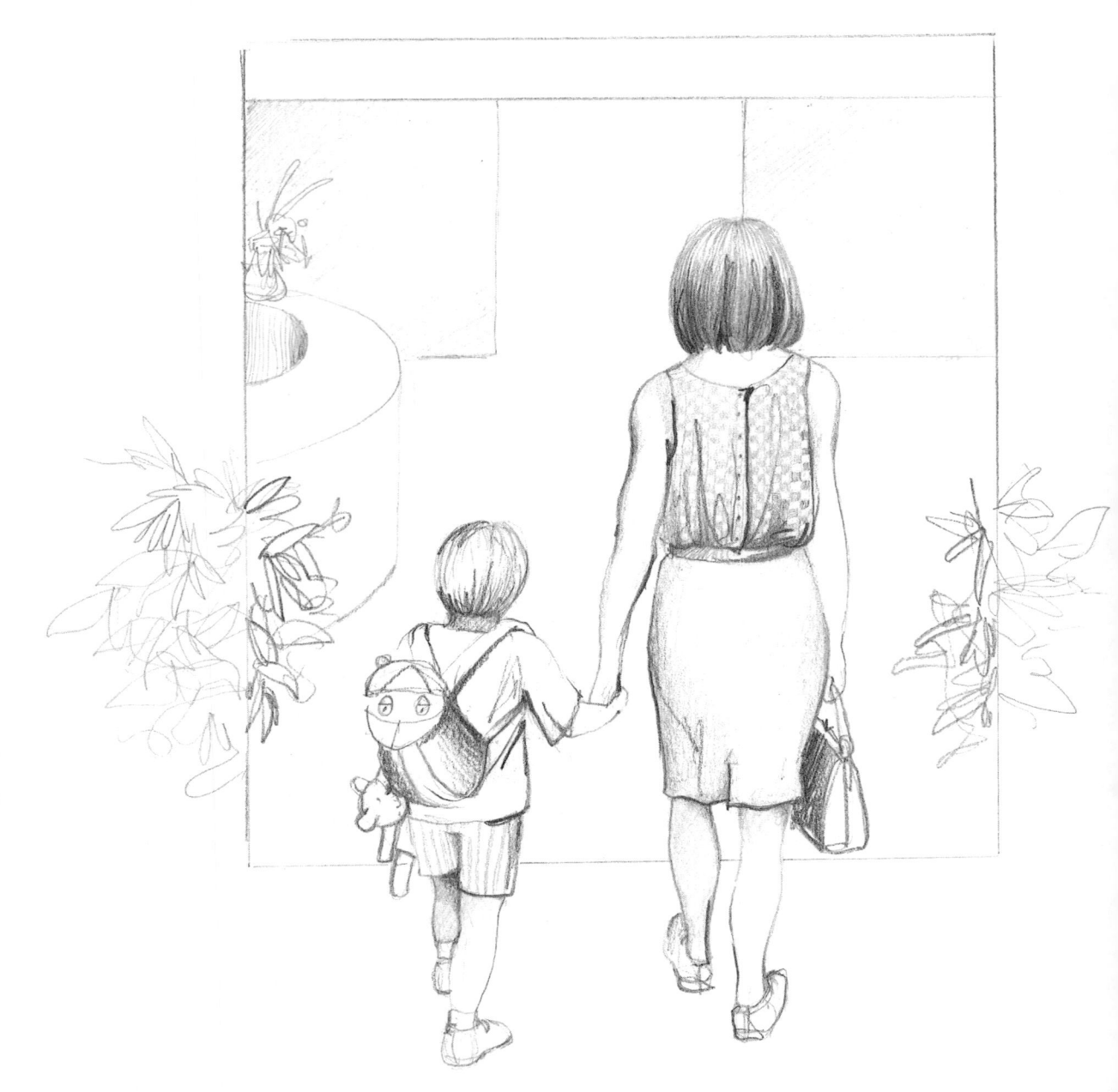

If in doubt, check with the hospital about what clothing and toilet items to take. Remember to take health insurance documents and any medicines the child may be taking, since they may need to be continued while he is in hospital.

When you go to the ward the nurse should be told about any special names, words or signs the child uses, for example, what he says when he wants to go to the toilet. You should also mention any food or activity that he especially likes or dislikes. If parents wish to bring in any special food for their child, this should always be discussed first with the nurse. Make certain that any food or medicine allergies are clearly noted in his records and on the bed.

What Happens After Admission

After all the formalities are completed your child will be changed into his bedclothes, weighed, a sample of urine collected and his temperature taken. He will be seen by a resident doctor and nurse, when a history is taken. You will be asked to sign consent for any proposed operation or treatment and you should not leave until this has been done. Make sure you understand what is to be done and any likely risks or complications of tests and treatments. If you're uncertain, ask the doctor to explain again or in more detail.

Special tests may now start. These might include blood tests, and will mean finger pricks or needles. No-one likes having needles. We know they hurt and a child should never be told they don't. However, the sting from the needles is only momentary and although children often cry, you can be sure they get over the hurt very quickly.

Living in and Visiting

Parents should spend as much time as possible with their child, helping with feeding, washing and playing with him. Brothers and sisters should visit. The child in hospital enjoys seeing them and it reassures brothers and sisters that all is going well.

Babies and young children are particularly upset if they are separated from their mothers, and living in at the hospital is often helpful to minimise the stress and aid recovery. Hospitals can usually accommodate parents, and this should be discussed with the staff before night-time when staff numbers are fewer.

A child who is having an operation needs his parents to be with him on that day, both before the operation and when he wakes up.

Children often cry when parents visit and this is a natural way of showing their feelings with someone safe and familiar. Children who are not visited by their family often become depressed and withdrawn; this is a much more disturbing sign than a few tears. If you can't visit regularly ask if the hospital has any scheme where volunteers might sit with your child and give him the one to one attention that nurses rarely have the time to give.

When parents leave their child to go home it's important to say good-bye even though the farewell may be upsetting for both parent and child. The child will be frightened and confused if parents just disappear. If parents are sure when they will return they should tell their child, but

A child who is having an operation needs his parents to be with him
▼▼▼

Going to hospital

When you leave, always tell a nurse who can comfort your child if he is upset
▼▼▼

they mustn't make impossible promises. It's helpful to some very young children if parents leave something which belongs to them, such as a scarf or handkerchief, to reassure the child that they will return. When you leave, always tell a nurse who can then be available to comfort your child if he is upset.

OPERATIONS AND ANAESTHETICS

Local anaesthesia is rarely used alone for operations on children, except for some older children who can understand and co-operate. This is not possible with younger children, and because of this and to avoid disturbing and frightening them, a general anaesthesia is usual. Children are normally told they will be 'put to sleep'. It's important that they be given a simple explanation that they can understand. They need to know that the anaesthetist can keep them asleep until it's time for them to wake up and that it's not possible for them to wake up too early while the operation is still taking place.

Following this the child is taken to the operating area. Being accompanied by a parent is very helpful but there is often a point of separation before anaesthesia is commenced. It's sometimes possible in special circumstances for parents to be present at the start of an anaesthetic. However, many anaesthetists prefer the parents and child to separate a little while before anaesthesia is started. This time of separation is often the hardest time for both parent and child and it's now that the parent should be most reassuring and tell the child they will be waiting afterwards when the child wakes up.

Anaesthesia is commenced either by an injection using a needle or by blowing anaesthetic gases over the child's face. Modern anaesthetic agents act much more quickly and are much more pleasant with fewer side-effects. Parents should never promise that the anaesthesia will be given in any particular way — this decision must be left to the anaesthetist and sometimes circumstances may necessitate a particular type of induction or a change in plans.

At the end of the operation the patient is normally sent to a recovery ward to wake up from the anaesthetic. He may have fluids running into his veins or be given oxygen by a mask. If this is likely to be so, the child and parents should be warned beforehand so it won't come as a surprise.

It is very helpful for the parents to be present as soon as possible after the child is returned to the recovery ward and be present when he wakes up. Being nursed by Mum is probably the best comfort there is. However, all children should be given pain-killing drugs when needed as there is no need for a child to suffer unnecessarily. Older children will be given the option of controlling their own pain-killing drugs.

Day-stay surgery

There is a growing trend for minor surgery to be done on a 'day-stay' basis. This means that the child is brought to hospital in the morning, has his operation and goes home on the same day after being checked by his doctor. A wider range of surgery is now undertaken on a day-stay basis.

For day-stay patients, a list of instructions is given about appropriate feeding and other preparations. It's important to carefully read these instructions and follow them exactly. It's equally important for parents to understand what they need to do after going home and to have a contact phone number should they need advice and help.

Colds and skin rashes

A problem that confronts many parents whose child is going to hospital for an operation is the common cold. Anaesthetists are reluctant to give anaesthetics to children who are in the acute stages of a cold because complications may occur. These include a severe form of croup or even pneumonia. Parents themselves are usually aware when their child is getting over a cold and anaesthesia and surgery at this stage is usually safe. Many children, especially those with adenoid problems, always have a blocked up nose and a cough. If your child is always like this, there is normally no reason why the anaesthesia and operation should be postponed.

If your child develops a skin rash or other symptoms you should always advise your doctor, since under certain circumstances it may be necessary to postpone the operation. If your doctor or the anaesthetist decides it is better to defer the operation, even though the child has been admitted to hospital, it's in the child's best interest. It's always disturbing to have to go through it all again, but it's much safer to do this than to run the risk of some unnecessary complication occurring.

If you're in doubt as to whether it's safe for an operation to proceed, get in touch with your doctor before you go to the hospital or ring the hospital for advice.

Being nursed by Mum is probably the best comfort there is
▼▼▼

Loose teeth

Since loose teeth may be dislodged and inhaled or swallowed during anaesthesia, it is important that they are mentioned to your doctor during a pre-operative visit or after arrival at hospital.

Physiotherapy

Physiotherapy means treatment by physical means, such as exercise, massage and heat
▼▼▼

Physiotherapy means treatment by physical means, such as exercise, massage and heat. It now forms a very important part of the treatment of many diseases in childhood. It's possible to undertake physiotherapy on children of any age from the newborn period onwards. Since physiotherapy often needs to be continued for long periods, it's important to involve the parents in the treatment so that they may understand what is being done, help in the physiotherapy and continue to carry out the treatment after the child returns home.

Physiotherapy is particularly helpful in the treatment of chest diseases, orthopaedic (bone) conditions, and diseases of the nervous system. Properly performed physiotherapy is a much more effective means of clearing secretions and giving treatment in such diseases as pneumonia and cystic fibrosis, than the old traditional cough mixtures.

Among the most common neurological conditions requiring physiotherapy are cerebral palsy and spina bifida. Sometimes head injuries or brain infections can leave a child with a permanent physical handicap. Such children will require physiotherapy as an early and continuing part of their management, and in such cases the parents can often contribute a great deal to the wellbeing and progress of their child by learning to undertake most of this physical treatment at home.

The rehabilitation should start at an early stage. The child needs to be stimulated as much as possible and must learn what normal movements feel like. The parents must be taught how to handle, carry, bathe, dress and play with their child in such a way that he is given every opportunity to behave and feel as normal as possible. It's important to maintain as normal a life as possible with the rest of the family and friends. Other children must be allowed to be the centre of attention sometimes to reassure them that they are loved as much as the sick brother or sister.

Plaster casts and splints are used both for support and for immobilisation. Some children need to be fitted with calipers to support weak or paralysed limbs and aid walking. Special splints are used in the management of congenital abnormalities of the joints and bones.

Hydrotherapy (treatment in warm water) is a useful way of mobilising children who suffer from muscle weakness or who have stiff and painful joints. The benefit results from the soothing effect of heat and the greater ease of movement in water which lessens the effects of gravity and makes muscle work easier.

Going home

When your child comes home after an operation you may be worried as to how much he can do safely. Ask your doctor about any limitation of physical activity and when it's safe for your child to have a bath. Remember that it's sometimes easier to rest a young child when he is up rather than being kept in bed.

Children recover much more quickly than adults. Those having day-stay surgery are often walking and playing the next day. If they need any medicine for pain or other discomfort, paracetamol mixture is usually adequate. But if in doubt, always consult your doctor.

Unfortunately, complications can occasionally arise following any operation. If there is any bleeding, persistent or increasing pain, temperature or any other problem after the child has come home, contact your doctor or the hospital without delay.

Your child may take time to settle down after he's been to hospital even though he's pleased to be home. Young children may be particularly upset by the experience and may become more babyish and demanding. They may have bad dreams, go off their food or regress in their behaviour such as wetting the bed again.

Changes in behaviour are common and you can help by being patient and understanding. Bad dreams, fear of the closed door or of the dark, and bed-wetting are all signs of anxiety and your child needs reassurance that he's safe and that his normal activities will begin again.

Parents should never punish their child for these relapses to more infantile behaviour patterns but they should be understanding and supportive. Things will quickly settle down.

To summarise, although going to hospital, and particularly, anaesthesia and surgery, will always have some emotional effect on a child, with adequate and truthful preparation by parents, doctors and nurses, and by the participation of the parents in his whole hospital experience, the undesirable effects can be minimised.

It's sometimes easier to rest a young child when he is up rather than being kept in bed
▼▼▼

CHAPTER 10

CHILD SAFETY —HOW SAFE IS YOUR CHILD?

In Australia it's estimated that there are almost 500 accidental deaths each year. Most of these result from road traffic accidents; drowning is the second most common cause of death. Accidents now cause three times as many deaths in children as any single disease!

Children between the ages of one and five years are the high risk group because, at this age, they need constant supervision. They are particularly prone to falling and to cutting themselves. Almost two-thirds of all children's accidents happen in the home and nearly one-third on the roads. The most dangerous areas in the home are the backyard and the kitchen, the laundry and the bathroom.

We can reduce the chance of accidents to our children in several simple ways:

- Supervision and protection of the very young
- Safety education as children grow older
- Understanding how accidents happen and foreseeing dangerous situations
- Selective legislation to create safer home design, safer play areas and a safer environment for children
- Being fully informed about accident prevention; in that way lives could be saved and permanent disability and disfigurement could be avoided

If after reading this chapter you would like more information about accident prevention, write to the Child Safety Centre in your children's hospital, or to:

Kid Safe — the Child Accident
Prevention Foundation of Australia
c/- Royal Australasian
College of Surgeons,
Spring Street,
Melbourne Victoria 3000

FALLS

- Fit safety catches on upstairs windows.
- Use safety gates on stairways.
- Fit safety glass in low level glass doors.
- Install good lighting on stairways.
- Wipe up spilt liquids in the kitchen at once.
- Encourage children to put toys away after use.
- Fix loose or torn carpets.

CUTS

- Keep knives, scissors and razor blades safely away from young children.
- Make sure glass doors are clearly marked.
- Sweep up broken glass — never pick it up — and wrap it well before putting it into the garbage bin.
- Glass bottles are easily broken: use plastic bottles or cartons whenever possible.
- Make sure that tetanus immunisation is kept up to date.

BURNS AND SCALDS

- Never permit young children to play with matches.
- Always have properly guarded household heaters.
- Never leave a young child unattended near an open fire or in the kitchen or bathroom.
- Always check the temperature of bath water and run the cold water before the hot water.
- Never buy long nightdresses or dressing gowns: use tight fitting tracksuit design pyjamas and dressing gowns for your children.
- Always turn saucepans and frying pan handles inwards.
- Never allow the hot-water jug cord to dangle over the edge of the bench.
- Always use tablemats instead of tablecloths if you have young children.
- Never place cups or pots of hot tea or coffee near the edge of the table.
- Install an approved smoke detector.

POISONS

- Always put tablets and medicines away in a high, locked or childproof cupboard: best of all, have a child restraint medicine cupboard. Each state has a Poisons Information Centre who can give you details, their number is in the emergency section of the phone book.
- Don't keep leftover tablets or medicines — get rid of them safely.
- Never store sink or oven cleaners under the sink where your small child can get to them.
- Keep household cleaners,

Children between the ages of one and five years need constant supervision ▼▼▼

detergents, bleaches and pesticides locked up: never store them with food.
- Always keep petroleum products and paint cleaners in their original containers; never store them in soft drink bottles.

INHALED AND INGESTED FOREIGN BODIES

- Young children like to put small objects in their mouths. Never give a child under five years nuts or small objects to eat or play with. Peanuts are the most commonly inhaled foreign body.
- If your child coughs and chokes suddenly or starts to wheeze, she could have inhaled a foreign body. Do not slap her on the back — take her straight to your doctor or ring your local hospital for advice.

ELECTRICAL SAFETY

- Obtain an inspection of the electrical system of your home from a qualified electrician.
- Never permit your child to play with power points.
- Turn off power points and unplug appliances when you're not using them.
- Fit safety plugs to all power outlets.

- Keep cords of toasters, jugs and appliances out of the reach of young children.
- Replace frayed cords and broken plugs promptly.

SAFETY IN THE BACKYARD

- Plan a safe playing area for your child; it should be fenced off from the road, carport and the driveway. For children up to the age of one, a portable playpen is a great help.
- Keep garden tools, the motor mower, pesticides, kerosene, paints and petrol in a locked shed in the garden. Better still, have a childproof cupboard for dangerous substances — not only for medicines.
- Take care not to plant poisonous shrubs if you have young children. Many common garden plants such as diffenbachia (a foliage plant) and oleander are poisonous if eaten. Others like the hybrid grevilleas cause allergic dermatitis.
- Never let children stand nearby if you are using a motor mower or edge trimmer.
- Make sure children are wearing shoes if they are playing in the garden.
- Never let children run holding a stick, or with anything in their mouth.

Plan a safe playing area for your child
▼▼▼

132   Your Child

WATER SAFETY

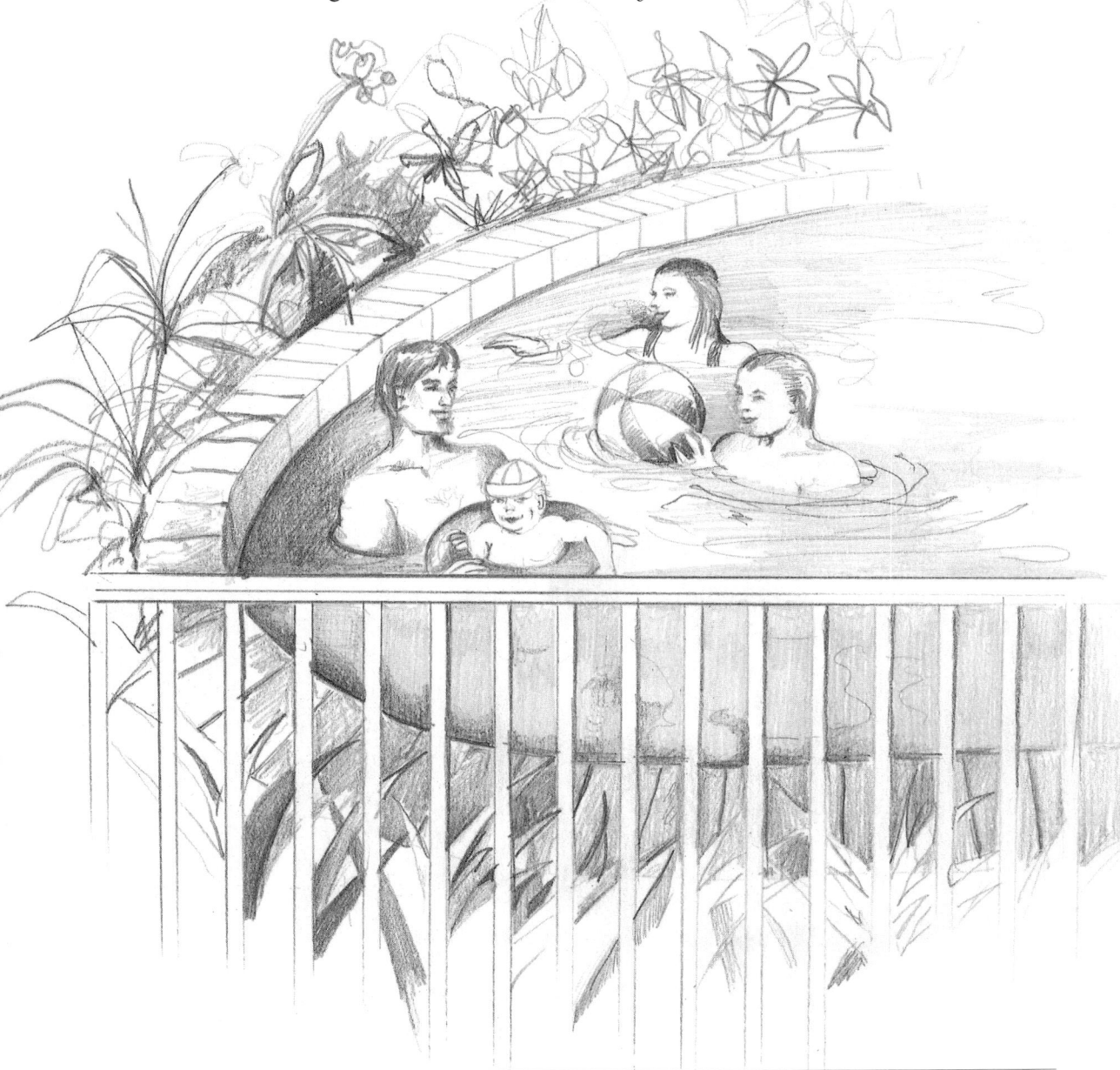

Around the world drowning is either the second or third most common cause of death in childhood. Not surprisingly, drowning is more common in countries where the climate is warm. It's interesting to compare the incidence of drowning in England and Australia. Between 50 and 100 children die from drowning each year in Britain while over 100 die each year in Australia, with a total population only just over one quarter of the United Kingdom. Most child drownings in Australia occur in home swimming pools, in marked contrast to Britain where drownings are more evenly divided between rivers and lakes, the sea and home pools.

Never allow children to swim alone or without the supervision of a responsible adult ▼▼▼

- Never leave your child alone or unsupervised near the water: remember that small children can drown in very shallow pools.
- Make sure your pool is enclosed by approved fencing with a self-closing gate: drownings rarely occur in properly fenced pools.
- Teach your child to swim but don't let this be a licence to drown: never allow children to swim alone or without the supervision of a responsible adult.
- Make sure there is a non-slip surface around the pool.
- Always make sure there is something that will float near the pool such as a coil of rope, a ball or a li-lo. It is always safer to throw something to anyone in difficulties — don't jump in.
- All members of the family should be taught mouth-to-mouth resuscitation and external cardiac massage.
- Ensure that pool chemicals are stored safely out of the reach of young children.
- Diving into shallow water can cause serious injury — concussion or even permanent paralysis: spinal injuries from diving, surfing and waterskiing occur more often than in any other sport.

SUNBURN AND HEAT EXHAUSTION

- The harmful short-term effects of sunburn and its long-term role in causing skin cancers are now widely recognised.
- Make sure infants and children wear a shady hat when they are not in the water.
- Use a suitable sunblock cream and reapply frequently even though the label says that it's waterproof.
- Take a shade umbrella and some cool drinks with you.
- Encourage children to wear T-shirts to reduce the risk of severe sunburn and don't spend too long in the hot sun, especially early in the summer season.

BARBECUES AND INCINERATORS

- Never leave children unsupervised if the barbecue or an incinerator is alight.
- Never throw flammable liquids, such as petrol, onto a barbecue to make it burn more quickly: use firelighters, kindling or paper.
- Dress little girls in tight-fitting clothes, such as jeans, rather than full skirts, for a barbecue.

- Never throw pressure-pack cans on a barbecue or incinerator; they will explode.
- Make sure the barbecue or incinerator is out when you leave it and that there are no matches left around for children to play with.
- Be sure that firelighters and any other flammable agents are put away well out of the reach of children.
- Always observe bushfire regulations and if there is no barbecue built, clear the ground around any you make yourself.

GUNS

Airguns are not toys. It is in fact illegal to give a child an airgun. Airguns are dangerous and potentially lethal. Airgun pellets can penetrate the skull or chest and abdomen, and deaths have occurred from such injuries. Airguns can also cause serious injury to the eyes.

- Regard all guns as possibly loaded.
- Never point a gun at another person.
- Keep ammunition in a separate place from the locked up gun.
- Be especially careful when cleaning your rifle and when climbing through fences with it.

PEDESTRIAN SAFETY

- Teach your child to understand the red, amber and green traffic lights and to obey them; teach her the 'walk' and 'don't walk' signs; teach her to use pedestrian crossings whenever possible and to cross in the company of an older child or adult. A child can understand all this at three years of age.
- Never allow your child to ride scooters or tricycles on the road.
- Teach your child the rules of the road as soon as she is old enough to understand them.
- Make sure your child wears clothing that is easily seen by an approaching motorist, particularly in wet weather and at sunset: raincoats should be bright yellow or orange.
- Never let children play on a street that is used by traffic: if there isn't a backyard to play in, take them to the park.

BICYCLE SAFETY

- Young children, under the age of nine years, should not be allowed to ride in traffic.
- Your child should not be given a bicycle until she knows the rules of the road.
- The most serious bicycle injuries are head injuries: insist

A child can understand basic road safety rules at three years of age
▼▼▼

Child safety...

that your child wears an approved cycle helmet whenever she is riding her bicycle.
- Children should wear conspicuous clothing when on the roads.
- Ensure that their bicycle is fitted with rear and front lights that work properly.

ROAD SAFETY

Children must be securely restrained in a car. Have seat belts fitted suitable to the age of your child. For young children you can obtain suitable belts to restrain bassinettes and child seats or booster seats approved by the Standards Association.

The safest place for your child is in the back seat properly restrained.

- Make sure you know exactly where your child is when you back the car out of the garage.
- Never leave your child unattended in a car: a child or an animal left in the car on a warm summer day can rapidly develop heatstroke and serious illness; even death may occur.
- Never leave matches or anything dangerous in the glove box; your child will find them — remember that the cigarette lighter still works when the ignition is turned off.
- Children can release the handbrake if they are alone in the car, even for a very short time, possibly with disastrous results.

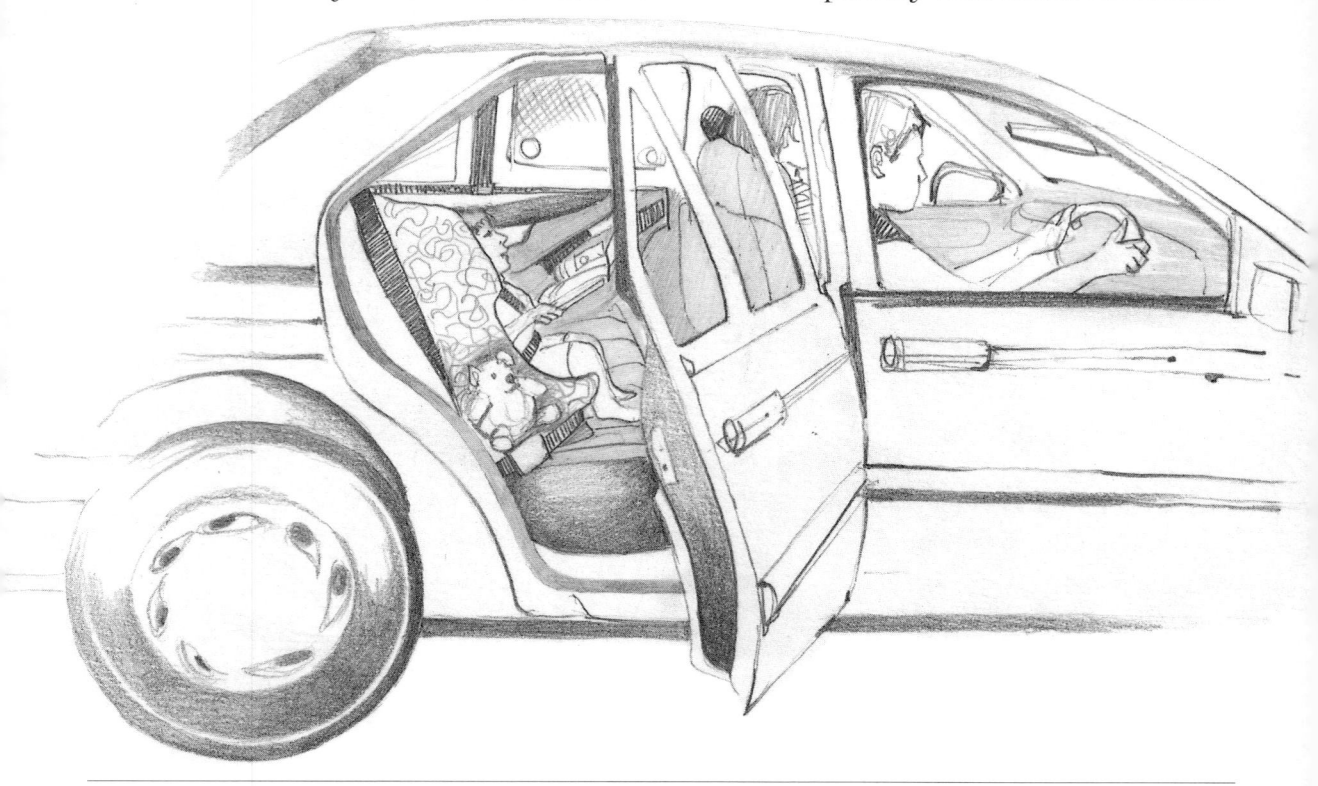

What to do in an Emergency

General

- Do not give anything to eat or drink when your child has had an accident in case she needs an anaesthetic when she gets to hospital.
- Do not move a child with a suspected neck or back injury.
- All head injuries are potentially serious — seek medical advice.
- If a child is unconscious, watch the airway — turn her face down or keep the chin firmly forward.
- Most bleeding will stop with direct pressure: then apply a firm pad and bandage.

Cuts and falls

- A firm bandage controls most bleeding: a tourniquet is rarely necessary and can be dangerous unless expertly applied.
- Seek medical advice without delay if it's more than a minor cut, if there is any loss of movement or function in a limb, continuous pain or swelling, any loss of consciousness, continuing or increasing drowsiness, or any vomiting, pallor or shock.

Burns and scalds

- Wrap the child in a rug, blanket, or a coat to put out the flames.
- With a scald, immediately apply plenty of cold water — iced if possible. Wrap the child in a clean sheet and go straight to the hospital. Do not apply any ointment or other substance.

Poisons

Call the Poisons Information Centre or your local hospital for urgent advice. If your child has swallowed a caustic like sink or oven cleaner or paint stripper, do not induce vomiting. Give her some milk to drink and go straight to the nearest hospital. If possible take the container from which your child has obtained the poisons or drugs with you so that the exact content of the product or the poison can be ascertained.

Do not give anything to eat or drink when your child has had an accident
▼▼▼

CHAPTER 11

SOME SPECIAL FAMILY SITUATIONS

SEPARATION AND DIVORCE

When separation is necessary, great care must be taken not to use the children as pawns in a game of mutual recrimination. In the arguments that may continue after divorce, wrangles over money and children are very common. Both parents should resolve not to embroil the children in their mutual conflict.

As with other stressful experiences, the ill effects on any particular child cannot be foretold accurately and will depend on the child's age, personality, intelligence and level of social development. Understandably, children will feel torn in their loyalties and have feelings of guilt about the separation of their parents. Care must be taken not to add to the child's feelings of conflict by one parent blaming or speaking disparagingly about the other. Whenever feasible, children should be given the opportunity of retaining loyalties to both parents.

Living arrangements should be designed for the child's benefit and depend on individual circumstances. It's usually preferable for children to live with their mother. However, access arrangements should be flexible and preferably carried out as a result of mutual agreement in which the wishes of the children have been taken into account. The rigid visiting schedules frequently laid down by the courts can become a burden and a frustration to parents and children alike. It will obviously be disruptive if the father poses as the 'nice guy', providing entertainment and goodies during the time he has access to the children, while the mother gains the reputation of being the mean one because she has to maintain discipline and exercise realistic restrictions at home.

SINGLE PARENTS

The child may be without a father because of death, divorce or because a mother chose to bring the baby up herself. The absence of a father makes a profound difference to a child, although with understanding, care and consideration such children can and do grow up to be normally adjusted people. It's important, however, that the mother doesn't allow her affection to make her child too dependent upon her to the exclusion of other healthy and normal associations that the child may make. The child, as he grows, needs some form of father substitute and this needs to have some permanence about it. Sometimes this can be provided by a grandfather, another male family relative or old family friend, provided they can form a sympathetic relationship with the child and see him fairly regularly.

In the case of the motherless child, there are similar problems but also additional difficulties. In most cases, the father will have a full-time job and will necessarily have to delegate the care of his children to somebody else during the day. He should make every effort to be with his children as much as possible after work until bedtime and at weekends. Because of the close and intimate relationship that normally exists between a mother and child, a mother substitute is even more difficult to find than a suitable father substitute. Today, more fathers who are single parents choose to leave work and become a house parent.

In many cases remarriage will occur. In this situation the stepmother or stepfather must understand that he or she has a particularly difficult task which will require tact, sympathy and understanding. This is particularly so if the natural mother or father is still alive and seeing the children regularly.

What all single parent families need is support: support in the emotional, social and material spheres. When this support is not forthcoming from other members of the family or friends, it must be sought through social agencies, religious or community groups or organisations such as 'Parents Without Partners'.

All single parent families need support in the emotional, social and material spheres
▼▼▼

STEP FAMILIES

There is a tendency for divorces in Australia to occur earlier in a marriage than they used to. This means that children in broken families tend to be younger and the separating parents younger as well. The result of course is that remarriage is more likely.

Luckily coping with and accepting a new parent seems to be easier for younger children than older children, especially teenagers.

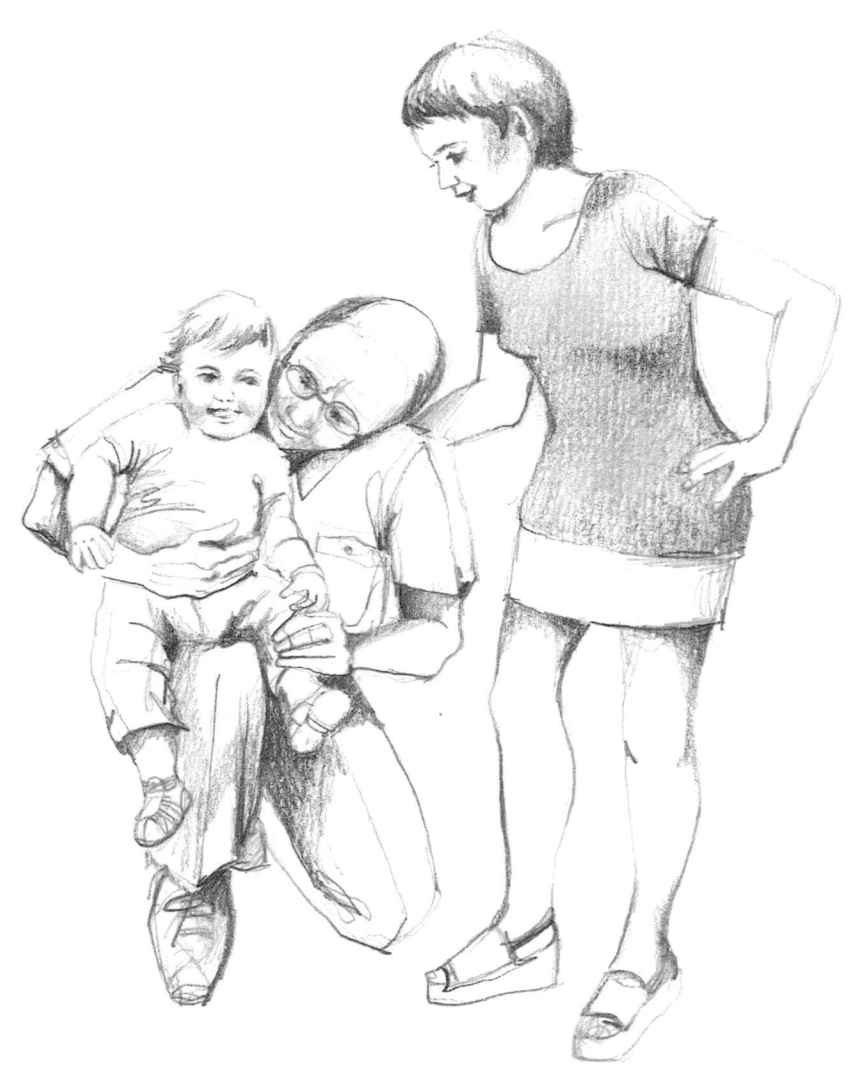

There is a real sense of loss felt by the affected children even though they may see both parents regularly. There is often a loss of financial status with both sides of a family having to make do with less.

There will always be the temptation on the part of a foster parent to buy favour with presents or to be less strict, but it is important to be true to your normally held views on discipline.

Step parents tend to think of the problems they face without considering the bewildering emotions that a child has when needing to be loyal to his natural parents and yet being fair to the foster parent.

The birth of a new baby by either the parent with custody or by the other parents presents another threat of lost affection or of jealousy. Remembering how a child may feel will go a long way to meeting his needs.

WORKING PARENTS

It is now very common for both parents to be working. In many cases the reason is purely economic, but in others both husband and wife are pursuing careers which they are reluctant to forsake. Mother will, of course, have to stop working late in pregnancy and for a certain length of time after baby arrives, but the question then arises as to whether she will stay at home with her child or resume her career. In a modern society both father and mother have an equal right to an outside career and an equal responsibility for child care. It's important, therefore, that they give careful consideration to their respective roles once they have a family. Ideally, this discussion should have taken place before a family is contemplated. Some parents take it in turn to pursue a career or to look after the children. Today almost any option is socially acceptable.

The way in which a child's emotional needs are met during the first two or three years of his life will have a lasting effect on subsequent emotional development. Therefore, whenever possible, a mother should devote a substantial amount of her time to her child during this very important phase. This is not necessarily inconsistent with a career. If at all possible, a mother should be prepared to devote full-time care and attention to her infant during the first four to six months to enable the intimate bonding relationship between her and her child to be fully established. Then, if she wishes to resume a career, there are some alternatives. In certain professions it may be possible to work from home. Others, such as nurses or workers in the service industry, can often arrange their working hours so they can spend most of the day with their baby, with an appropriate substitute to cover the other hours. It may be possible to work part-time or in broken shifts to allow adequate time to be spent with the baby, at least until he is old enough to attend kindergarten. Then, of course, the father can be the carer.

The choice of a suitable parent substitute requires considerable care. An understanding grandmother may seem to be a satisfactory solution, but remember: firstly, she may find it a strain at her age to satisfy the demands of an active young child and secondly, it's difficult to 'sack' her if this doesn't turn out to be a satisfactory arrangement. If you have to leave your child in the care of someone else it's important to try to provide continuity of care; a succession of mother substitutes will only confuse baby and induce a sense of insecurity and uncertainty. After continuity of care, the most important qualities to look for are

Some parents take it in turn to pursue a career or to look after the children
▼▼▼

Some special family situations 141

commonsense, affection, self-reliance and understanding.

Even if your mother substitute turns out to have all these qualities in full measure — and she will be a pearl beyond price if she does! — make sure that you spend sufficient time in caring for your child to avoid a major transfer of her dependence and affection to the mother substitute. Otherwise this can create problems later on when the inevitable separation occurs.

Economic and social considerations may make it essential for you to work and rely on a day care centre. The day care centre should preferably be on the way from your home to work so that it is easy for you to drop your child off and pick him up.

It's important to love the adopted child for his own qualities ▼▼▼

ADOPTION

With the fall in birth rate and the increasing availability of abortion, the number of children available for adoption has decreased markedly. Many couples who, for various reasons, are unable to have children of their own want to adopt a baby. The relevant government agency has definite requirements which must be met before you can proceed to adoption. These requirements relate mainly to your being able to provide a satisfactory home, to have a stable marriage and to be both mature enough and suitable in every way to care for and bring up a child.

Prospective parents have a variety of reasons for wanting to adopt a child. The most common reason is that they are unable to have a child of their own. In other cases, for humanitarian or social reasons, they may decide to adopt the child of a relative or friend or a child from a developing country. Other parents decide to take on the care of a child with some physical, developmental or emotional handicap.

In some cases, prospective parents or the government agency decide that it is preferable for a child to be fostered rather than adopted. Sometimes adoption is delayed in a child with a medical problem until the child's progress can be adequately evaluated or until the suitability of the placement is tested.

If you already have a child or children of your own, you should consider the potential problems if you adopt another child, and this should always be carefully discussed with an experienced paediatrician or social worker before proceeding.

The question of adoption after the death of a child is also something that needs very careful consideration and expert advice to ensure the adoption is not an attempt to replace the lost child. It may be wise to allow an interval of time so that you can work out your grief before proceeding to adoption.

Inevitably some comparison will be made, but it's important to love the adopted child for his own qualities and to carefully avoid any comparison between two children. Parents who lose children often have an idealised memory of the child they have lost and it will be impossible for the adopted child to measure up to this.

It is essential that an adopted child be told that he is adopted. If you fail to tell him you can be quite sure that some 'well meaning' person will, and this can be a very disturbing blow for the child. The best way to handle this, from a very early age, is to allow the fact to come into normal conversation and discussion with the child and with friends and acquaintances in the presence of your child. There's no need to go to the other extreme and exaggerate the importance of the matter. It should just come to be accepted as a natural part of the life of that family. It is, of course, quite appropriate to explain to your child, when he is old enough to understand, that you chose him especially because it was impossible to have a baby of your own.

It's preferable for the adopting parents to have no contact or continuing association with the natural parents. The government agency arranges for appropriate investigation and medical examination prior to adoption, but in most cases it's unwise for other information about the natural parents to be either sought or given. Your adopted child will gain security from the knowledge that you love him and that you want to continue to care for him as an integral part of your family. Many states now have laws permitting adopted people to access information about their natural parents, and parents who have adopted out their children access to information about the adopting family. Most laws, however, provide privacy provisions if any party does not wish such information to be given out.

> *It is essential that an adopted child be told that he is adopted*
> ▼▼▼

Some special family situations 143

CHAPTER 12

A LOOK INTO THE FUTURE

HEALTH NEEDS DURING ADOLESCENCE

Adolescence is the period of life between being a child and being an adult. During this time of growth, many changes occur physically, emotionally, psychologically and socially.

The psychological changes required before adult maturity is reached may be summarised as follows:

- Realisation of one's own identity
- Achievement of independence from parents
- Recognition and acceptance of one's sexuality
- Establishment of a pattern of philosophy for living and for relating to others
- Decisions about the future in terms of further education and career
- These will happen at a time and in a sequence that is different from adolescent to adolescent. Normal people can show a vast range of differences.

When an adolescent becomes ill, particularly if the illness is a serious or prolonged one, it may be harder for her to achieve these changes. She should be helped to be independent by being given the opportunity to tell the doctor the medical details herself, to participate in decisions about treatment and appointment times, and be given some responsibility for herself and her illness. Confidentiality should be maintained as much as possible. Medical appointments and hospital admissions should take her schooling into consideration. The effects of illness or disability on her attractiveness to her friends and peers, her sexuality, future parenthood and her future vocation, should be discussed. These considerations will help to make an illness a positive experience for the adolescent if she continues to have the loving concern of her family and the understanding of her professional advisers.

Common medical problems of adolescence include acne, overweight, menstrual period irregularities, problems of growth in height, and sexual maturity either too early or too late. Girls are particularly concerned about being too tall and boys about being too short. Sports injuries are fairly common, especially for boys.

Teenagers with diabetes, epilepsy and other chronic medical illness can have particular problems when growing up. Those with mental or physical handicaps need special consideration by schools and medical care givers. Medical conditions that have been stable for years can suddenly go wrong. Keeping to diets and taking medicines can assume major difficulties overnight.

PUBERTY

Puberty refers to the period of rapid growth when sexual development and other physical changes take place. The time at which puberty begins varies greatly. In general, the first signs of puberty appear in girls at about ten or eleven years and in boys at about eleven or twelve. Adolescents often worry if their development is out of step with their friends, and they may need to be reassured about the wide range of 'normal' development. Puberty also varies with race with some groups maturing earlier than others.

PUBERTY IN GIRLS

The first visible sign of puberty in a girl is growth of her breasts. One breast may develop before the other or grow faster. This is nothing to worry about. Usually the differences will disappear or be barely noticeable as puberty progresses. Occasionally breasts are too large, but more commonly, girls worry that their breasts are too small. Breast shape and size does not affect ability to respond sexually or to produce milk, but an anxious teenager may be difficult to reassure at this age when her main concern is her physical attractiveness and being like her friends.

The commencement of periods is a dramatic event in a girl's life. By this time pubic hair will be present and there will have been an increase in height (the adolescent growth spurt). While periods may normally commence any time from nine to eighteen years, if they have not occurred by sixteen years it's wise to arrange a medical check up. For the first year or so periods are quite irregular in the amount of menstrual loss and in frequency, but will usually settle down to a regular cycle in time. Contrary to popular belief, pregnancy can occur at this time. As menstruation is a symbol of reaching womanhood and sexual maturity, it is most important that this should not commence as an unexplained, unexpected and

Puberty refers to the period of rapid growth when sexual development and other physical changes take place
▼▼▼

frightening experience. In this regard the attitudes and support of parents, family and friends are very important. Mothers often find it easier to talk to their daughters than fathers to their sons. It's better for the first explanations to be made in the family than for young people to hear incorrect information from school friends.

Puberty in boys

Boys start to develop a year or two later than girls, which is why at the end of primary school some girls look more like boys' grown-up sisters than their classmates. The first visible sign of puberty in boys is an enlargement of the testicles. This is followed by the appearance of pubic hair and growth of the penis. It may take several years for development to be completed. It's no fun for a boy to lag behind his mates in these events, and if there is no sexual development by about thirteen and a half years, a doctor should be consulted. Generally, no physical abnormality will be discovered, but for boys who are slow developers (delayed adolescence) reassurance and emotional support are often needed.

Some time after sexual development has begun, the first ejaculation of semen may occur. This is more or less equivalent in significance to the first period in girls, but less fuss is made about it. It may occur as a 'wet dream' and cause sticky pyjamas which is embarrassing if it's unexpected, or it may be the result of masturbation or self-stimulation. Despite all the old wives' tales, masturbation is a normal and totally harmless practice. Parents should not be concerned about it but should ensure that their son understands what is socially acceptable sexual activity in their community or family.

Another cause for embarrassment is the sudden appearance of an erection, occasionally at the most inappropriate time. The only thing to do is to try and think of other things or try to ignore it. Some breast enlargement in boys is also normal. There is often a tender lump beneath the nipple but this will soon go away. Another source of concern and embarrassment is a 'breaking voice' which may even persist during the latter stages of puberty. It is due to the development of the larynx or voice box which changes to produce the deeper voice of mature males.

Pimples and spots

Most teenagers have to cope with a nasty trick of nature — acne. The hormones which cause the changes of puberty also work on glands in the skin, making them produce more oil than is necessary. The oil gets stuck in

> *It may take several years for development to be completed*
> ▼▼▼

the pores, is stained by dirt to make a blackhead and when this gets infected by skin bacteria, a pimple results. There are effective treatments for acne. Teenagers should wash themselves frequently and try not to squeeze pimples. In time they simply go away, but if they don't, then a vitamin A related ointment is used. This medicine can also be taken by mouth in more severe cases. It is effective when given in the right dose, but persistent use of larger doses may be dangerous so always use these preparations as advised by your doctor. Sometimes your doctor may prescribe a low dose course of antibiotics.

Adolescent sexuality

Sexual attitudes and behaviour by young people today have changed. As adults we must adjust to this and try to understand it. Physiologically, adolescents now mature at an earlier age; psychologically they have a more difficult and challenging time and they live in a more permissive society than their parents.

What is sexuality?

On a superficial level, sex simply means the act of sexual intercourse or the physical contact between the sexual organs. Sexuality, however, is a complex concept. It includes all our feelings, relationships and qualities as sexual beings. For adolescents there is perhaps more confusion now than ever before. Male and female roles have become less clear-cut and we live in an era where unisex image and behaviour are acceptable and common. Teenagers often feel under pressure to make choices regarding their sexuality and frequently they are too emotionally immature to cope. They become further confused because adult society often appears vague about their own attitudes, beliefs and standards. This is made more difficult by the lack of a black and white distinction between hetero-sexuality and homosexuality. Understanding, tolerance and love are much more effective in helping young people discover themselves than psychiatrists and psychologists.

Sexual behaviour in teenagers

An adolescent developing his or her individual sexuality is faced with a number of options:

- To avoid sexual encounters
- 'Kiss and cuddle' only

Understanding, tolerance and love are effective in helping young people discover themselves
▼▼▼

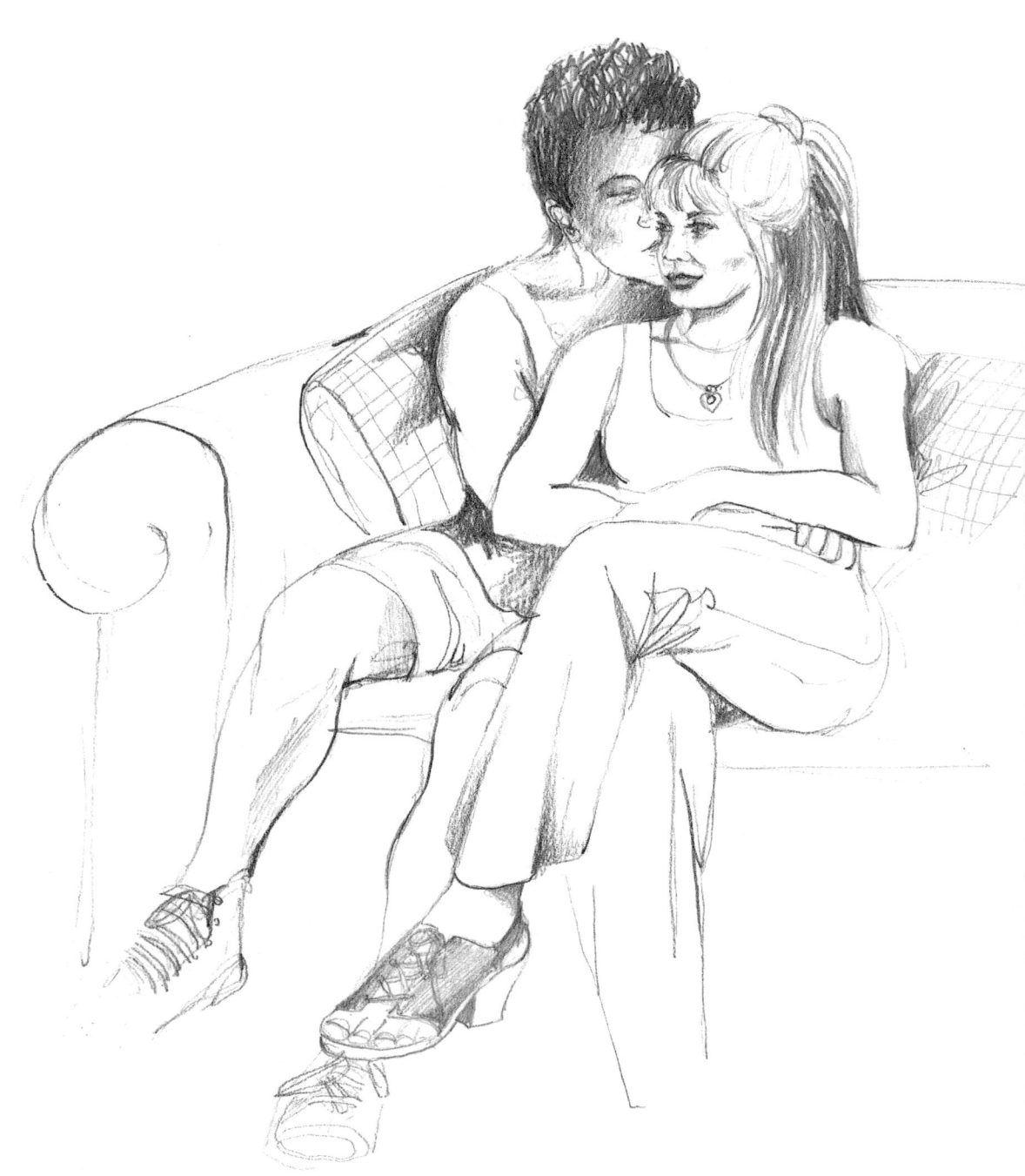

- To have sexual intercourse because of 'love'
- To be sexually promiscuous

There is evidence that the overall scene is changing. More adolescents are sexually active than in the past and are starting at a younger age. Surprisingly, sexually active young people are usually less knowledgeable than their 'inexperienced' peers.

There is a strong relationship between sexual ignorance and the increasing incidence of teenage pregnancy and venereal disease.

The advent of Human Immunodeficiency Virus or HIV and AIDS has made everyone more aware of the potential consequences of sexual play and intercourse and has promoted the use of condoms and safe sex. Putting aside any questions of morality, condoms and safe sex protect from AIDS, other venereal diseases and pregnancy.

Unfortunately, most teenagers don't know how to recognise symptoms of venereal disease and find treatment if they contract it, but hotlines and other anonymous advisory services have made help very much more accessible.

It's worth considering why sexually active young people rarely use effective contraceptives. This cannot be attributed to ignorance alone. One reason is the belief that sexual relations should be 'spontaneous and unplanned'. Contraceptives may be seen as too troublesome or inconvenient, or interfere with the pleasure of sex. Of course, some believe 'it cannot happen to me' or 'I am too young to fall pregnant'. A minority of girls who become pregnant deliberately plan to do so. Many are just unprepared and naive.

SOME OF THE HARMFUL CONSEQUENCES

For girls in particular, with their greater need for affection than boys, there is a danger of becoming emotionally involved more deeply than they can handle at their particular stage of maturity.

Pregnancy is a risk for sexually active teenage girls. The implications vary depending on whether the girl is at early, middle or late adolescence. At these various stages their knowledge, attitudes towards mothering, future plans and ability to cope will vary. For girls under seventeen years there are increased physical risks with pregnancy, with a greater chance of anaemia, prolonged labour and premature birth. Almost invariably there are emotional problems, disruption of educational and vocational plans and a greater risk for the baby.

Abortion, which in some States is readily available, is not without its problems. Depending on factors such as emotional maturity and family support, there may or may not be significant emotional disturbance associated with this. Studies have shown that girls who have had an abortion have a significant likelihood of a further unplanned pregnancy.

The majority of cases of venereal disease occur in young people aged from fifteen to twenty-four years. In boys, gonorrhoea, the most common type, usually causes a penile discharge and irritation. This means that it can be recognised

For girls under seventeen years there are increased physical risks with pregnancy
▼▼▼

early and treated. However, in many girls (and in some boys) it does not cause any symptoms. This is a particularly dangerous situation for girls, as an unrecognised infection can lead to later sterility. Girls who have symptoms usually experience pain in the lower part of the abdomen, a discharge from the vagina or, in more severe instances, can be quite ill with high fever and joint pains.

HIV infection may be completely asymptomatic for many years and in the sexually active teenager, this poses great dangers to their sexual partners. The use of condoms offers the greatest protection to all parties.

How can we help adolescents cope with their sexuality?

Although there is a pressing need for more and better sex education programs, there is a considerable amount that parents or concerned adults can do on an individual level. The following are simple guidelines.

- Give the adolescent credit for knowing something.
- Give her a chance to talk and ask questions — learn to listen!
- Display a sincere interest in her as an individual.
- Be honest with her, trust her.
- Respect her point of view.
- Be flexible.
- Provide knowledge on her level. Comic books and other literature about sex and safe sex are available from most youth health centres and the Family Life Movement.
- Actively engage her in the solution to her own problem.
- Provide a good role model for your teenager.

Some important facts teenagers should know

Sexual thoughts are normal. There is no need to feel guilty about socially unacceptable desires. Thoughts, images and fantasies cannot in themselves injure the individual. There is, of course, a distinction between thought and behaviour, and it's only for socially unacceptable behaviour that one must accept responsibility.

Homosexual thoughts and experiences are not often signs that an adolescent is becoming a homosexual — many boys and girls go through a stage of having these thoughts and experiences during adolescence, without being homosexual. If homosexual preference persists, young people should be helped to accept themselves without feeling guilty. There is no place for psychiatric treatment for what many now accept as part of the normal variation of human behaviour.

There is a pressing need for more and better sex education programs
▼▼▼

JUVENILE DELINQUENCY

Delinquency is basically a legal concept defined differently in different places. 'Juvenile delinquency' is a term usually applied to persons under sixteen or eighteen years of age who behave in a manner that is unlawful and punishable by law.

Delinquency has always existed but its reported incidence is rising. For many, delinquent behaviour actually begins in middle childhood or even earlier. Although more boys come to the attention of the authorities, the proportion of delinquent girls is increasing. Boys are more often involved in active or aggressive behaviour such as car thefts, joy-riding and burglary, whereas girls are more likely to be reported for running away from home, illicit sexual behaviour and because parents are unable to control them. More recently, girls seem to be becoming involved in more serious crimes and this is often related to drugs and their need to buy them.

The causes of delinquency are complex. It is thought, in part, to be due to changes in the structure of society. It may also be seen in some as a struggle to change the family unit or society. Delinquents tend to come more often from broken, disturbed or economically deprived homes with fragile family structures.

These young people are more likely to feel inadequate, emotionally rejected and frustrated in expressing themselves. They may not like, value or respect themselves and tend to be confused in their feelings and attitudes. They are more likely to be inconsistent and to be more attention-seeking than most teenagers. They also have difficulty forming close relationships with other teenagers. Generally speaking, the better a teenager gets on with her parents, the less likely she is to be delinquent in her behaviour. Although it is said that delinquency is more common in broken homes, this is not always the case. It is far more common in non-broken homes where there is mutual hostility, indifference or apathy and a lack of cohesiveness, than in broken homes where there is still cohesiveness, mutual affection and support. Inconsistency in discipline is thought to be a further factor.

Teenagers with these basic difficulties often have difficulty coping with the normal stresses of growing up. They may feel that explosive rebelliousness is the only way to find freedom. Belonging to a group organised around anti-social activity may be seen as a way to solve problems. It may also be used as a protest against the hypocrisy and double standards that the young person sees in adult society.

The better a teenager gets on with her parents, the less likely she is to be delinquent
▼▼▼

Parents concerned that their children or adolescents are showing signs of delinquent behaviour should seek early help from their local health centre or the Department of Community Services in their State, their doctor or a voluntary family agency.

Services designed for drug and alcohol problems exist in most areas
▼▼▼

DRUG USE BY ADOLESCENTS

Use of drugs by young people seems to many older people to characterise the lack of communication and the difference in values which may occur between the generations. Although the use of most drugs is increasing, and teenagers are using them at an earlier age, the majority who take drugs are simply experimenting. This is most likely if they are maintaining good relationships with family and friends and are continuing satisfactorily at school. The majority do not go on to hard drugs.

Our culture, however, is increasingly a drug-taking one. A young person is most likely to take drugs if her parents do, but the most important influence is that of friends. The highest rate of usage is where both friends and parents take drugs.

Heavy drug users, particularly multiple drug users and also problem drinkers, whose way of life is altered by their habit, are most likely to have acute and intense needs for which they are unable to gain relief in more acceptable, less destructive ways. They tend to be disadvantaged adolescents with emotional difficulties and profound disturbances in family relationships during development. These teenagers are likely to progress to the more dangerous drugs.

Services designed for drug and alcohol problems exist in most areas and are generally more helpful than conventional health services.

PREVENTION

Parents can help prevent young people getting 'hooked' in the following ways.

- Try to meet their children's emotional needs so that drugs don't become a substitute for the warmth, concern and security that they can give.
- Not always appear to be needing a drink or a smoke or a sleeping pill. Young people need to know that they do not have to drink, and that if they do, they should drink in a controlled and moderate way.
- Talk about drugs in a general way as they grow up. If evidence of drug taking is discovered, don't panic or lecture the teenager, but treat

her like an adult. Drug experimentation may not be serious and your reactions at crucial times are important.

Signs of drug use

These vary according to the drug used. Help should be sought for persisting unusual or deteriorating behaviour. For specific information or help in a difficult situation, ring the health educator or drug counsellor at your local community centre. They will be able to advise you about the many organisations both governmental and voluntary, where drug education, prevention and management programs are available. Advice given is confidential and no personal records are kept.

Normal Adolescent Behaviour

Parents can be puzzled and sometimes disturbed by normal adolescent behaviour.

Adolescence is a specific period in human development characterised by rapid and dramatic changes — physically, intellectually and emotionally — which may result in increased conflict with oneself and others. To become a mature adult involves achieving an appropriate degree of independence, a secure identity, a clear sexual identification, a suitable vocation and a place in society.

The best way to understand the progression of events is to consider adolescence in terms of three stages — early, middle and late.

The early adolescent with her rapidly developing body, often feels out of control and may be concerned about whether or not she is normal. There is usually a lot of rushing about, especially with friends of the same age and mostly the same sex. Early efforts to obtain emotional separation from parents may cause conflict at home. Daydreaming is normal and can be an additional cause of conflict and misunderstanding between parents and the adolescent.

In middle adolescence problems with parents often increase and the struggle for independence reaches its peak. The major goals at this stage are to be attractive, accepted and popular. This is the age of group activities. Teenagers tend to identify with adult heroes other than parents. They may be idealistic in outlook and as a result often feel misunderstood and rejected. A rich fantasy life is generally related to sexual situations or imagined great achievements.

By late adolescence a satisfactory degree of

Daydreaming is normal and can be an additional cause of conflict
▼▼▼

Teenagers need the support and understanding of mature adults
▼▼▼

independence is emerging and 'maleness' and 'femaleness' established. Often there'll be a special person of the opposite sex in the teenager's life, and these relationships are now more likely to involve mutual caring and responsibility. Intentions regarding vocation, mating and lifestyle are beginning to crystallise.

It's important to understand that rapid fluctuations characterise adolescence and your teenager may be happy and cheerful one minute and inexplicably miserable and sombre the next. Of course, growing up in today's confusing world is not easy and more than ever before, teenagers need the support, guidance and understanding of mature adults. They also need to be considered and respected as individuals. Oscar Wilde said:

Children begin by loving their parents
As they grow older they judge them;
Sometimes they forgive them.

Special Information for Emergencies

Keep a list of these phone numbers — they will save time and perhaps a life:

Your doctor

District hospital

Children's hospital

Your dentist

Ambulance

All-night chemist

Poisons Information Centre operates a 24 hour service. Call the appropriate number in your state or territory.

ACT	(06) 285 2852
NSW	(02) 692 6111
	008 25 1525
NT	(089) 228 842
QLD	(07) 253 8233
	008 17 7333
SA	(08) 204 6117
	008 18 2111
TAS	(002) 38 8485
	008 001400
VIC	0055 15678
WA	(09) 381 1177
	008 119244

For further advice and information on child safety, contact the Child Safety Centre on 692 6833 or write to them at PO Box 34, Camperdown NSW 2050. Or you can contact the National Safety Council of Australia on the following local numbers.

Sydney	(02)690 1555
Melbourne	(03)824 8822
Brisbane	(07)252 8977
Adelaide	(08)234 3034
Perth	(09)340 8509
Hobart	(002)23 2853
Northern Territory	(089)470 404

Write in the space below any other emergency numbers you may find applicable and keep this as your 'Emergency Directory'.

The publisher has made every effort to ensure that all contact details were correct when this book went to print.

If you are in any way associated with children you owe it to them, yourself and the community to be familiar with external cardiac massage, mouth-to-mouth resuscitation and what to do for choking. Your knowledge may save a life.

CHOKING

When an infant or small child is choking on food or an object, seek urgent medical advice; but if he is blue, unable to cry or losing consciousness, place him over your knee, face down, and slap him on the back of his chest.

For an older child, stand behind the child with your arms folded together over his upper abdomen, just under his rib cage, and give a firm quick squeeze. This will push air out of his lungs and up into the windpipe and so dislodge the foreign body.

EXTERNAL CARDIAC MASSAGE

Before commencing external cardiac massage you must be absolutely sure that the heart has ceased to beat.

The force exerted on the chest depends on the size of the patient.

1. Two fingers on the centre of the chest in the case of a baby, at the rate of 90 presses per minute.
2. Five fingers for a child up to five or six years old; 75 presses per minute.
3. The heel of one hand for a child from six to twelve years; 60 presses per minute.
4. The heels of both hands for a child over twelve years or an adult; 60 presses per minute.

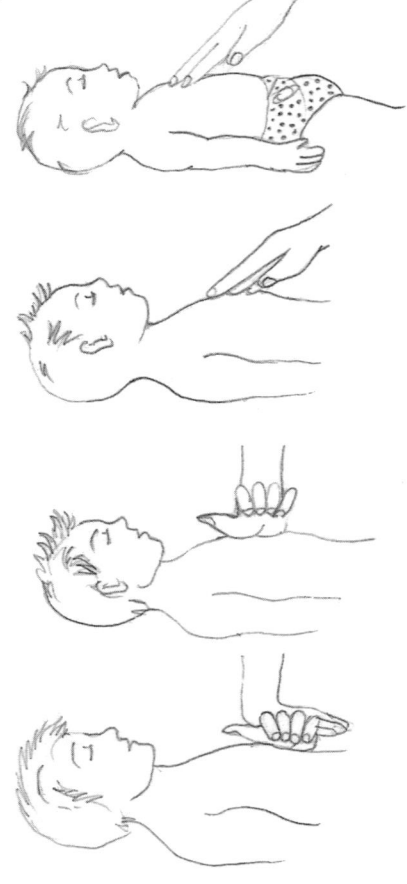

MOUTH-TO-MOUTH RESUSCITATION

Use 20 gentle puffs per minute for a baby, 15 breaths for a child and 12 for an adult. Try to continue resuscitation for at least one hour.

1. Lie the patient on his side and check mouth for foreign bodies.
2. Gently move patient onto back; place head and neck in position indicated to permit free passage of air.
3. Place fingers of one hand over nose to close off nostrils; continue to support neck with free hand.
4. Breathe into mouth and watch for stomach to rise as lungs fill with air.
5. Allow patient to exhale while you inhale.

With small children do not close nostrils with hand; breathe into both mouth and nose.

If you are alone, external cardiac massage and mouth-to-mouth resuscitation can be combined by doing 15 presses, 2 breaths, 15 presses, and so on.

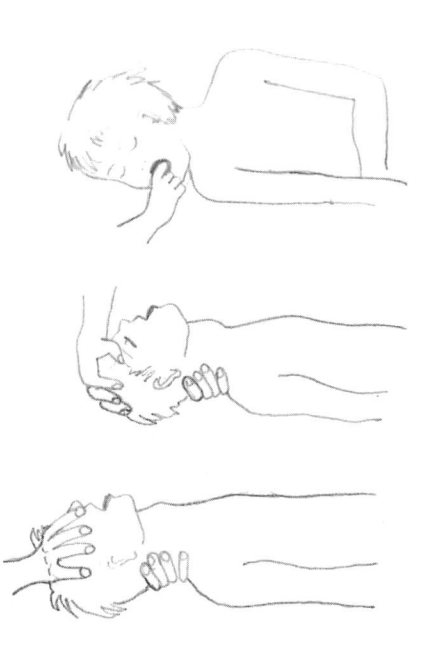

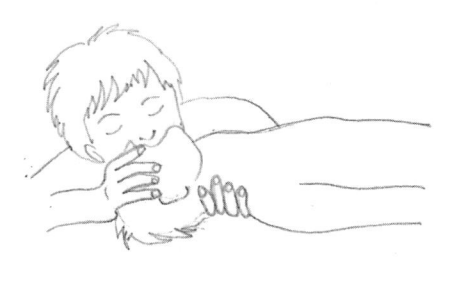

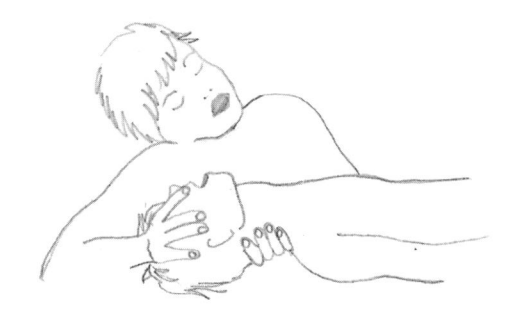

Special information

INDEX

abdominal pain 106
Aboriginal children,
　immunisation 50
abortion 149
accidents
　prevention 130-6
　what to do 137
acne 93-4, 146-7
adenoids 87
adolescents
　delayed adolescence 146
　delinquency 151-2
　drug use 152-3
　health needs 144-5
　normal behaviour 152-3
　puberty 145-7
　sexual activity 147-50
adoption 142-3
afterbirth 17
afternoon tea
　for toddlers 37
　weight reduction 39
aggression from siblings 23
AIDS 149
air travel 52-3
airguns 135
alcohol
　effect on breastfeeding 31
　teenagers 152
allergies 116
　eyes 90
amniocentesis 82, 112
amniotic fluid 17
anaesthetics 126-8
　explaining to child 123
anger
　siblings' 23
　tantrums 46, 61-3
animals 71
antibiotics 85, 87
anxiety, siblings' 23
appendicitis 106
appetite 38
arthritis 96
asthma 101-2, 116
astigmatism 89

baby
　brothers and sisters 22-3
　care 26-7
　clothes 28
　development 17-18
　father's role 22
　feeding 28-37
　first month 24-5
　grandparents 23-4
　hospitalisation 121
　loving 22
　malformations 111-14
　newborn 19-22
　relating to others 55
　relationship with mother 54-5
　skin problems 91-3
Baby Health Centres 26
baby-sitters 57-8

backyard safety 132
bad language 63-4
barbecue safety 134-5
bath
　after hospitalisation 129
　baby's 27
bed-wetting 47, 67
bedtime 60-1
behaviour problems 58-67
bicycle safety 135-6
bilingualism 44
birth
　baby at 19
　classes 16
　father at 54
　mother's reaction to baby 22
birthing units 16
birthmarks 94
bites 95
bladder
　control 47, 67
　problems 107-8
blindness 81
'blue babies' 112
boils 93
bonding
　father 22
　mother 54
　sick babies 113
bone problems 95-8
books 71, 73-4
bottle-feeding 30-1
bowed legs 49, 96
bowel
　see also stools
　control 47
　malformation 113
brain
　infections 128
　inflammation 100
　tumours 110
breakfast
　baby's 35
　for toddlers 37
　weight reduction 39
'breaking voice' 146
breast-feeding 28-30, 31-2
　building relationship with baby 54
breasts
　adolescent boys 146
　adolescent girls 145
　babies', at birth 20
　during feeding 31
　engorged 29
　size 31
breath holding 46, 63
breathing, noisy 86
bronchitis 86, 101
bronchodilators 102
broncho-pneumonia 101
brothers and sisters
　jealousy of baby 64
　response to new baby 22-3
burns
　preventing 131
　what to do 137
calipers 128
cancer 110-11
car sickness 52

car travel 52
　safety 136
cardiac massage 156
career 141
cats 71
cerebral palsy 128
cerebrospinal fluid 117
chest problems 101-3
chicken pox 100
choices, making 44-5
choking 156
chorionic villus sampling 82, 112
chromosomes 18
circumcision 108-9
cleft lip or palate 113-14
clothes, baby's 28
club foot 96
cochlear implantation 81
coffee 31
colds 85-6
　and surgery 127
colic 34, 59-60
colostrum 30
comforters 46, 59
concentration span 45
conception 17
condoms 149, 150
congenital malformations 111-14
conjunctivitis 89-90
constipation 103-4
contraceptives 149, 150
convulsions
　epileptic 118
　febrile 115
cot death 120
coughs 85-6
　whooping cough 100
cow's milk
　allergy 116
　formula feeding 30
cradle cap 20, 91
crime 151
crossed eyes 89
croup 86
crying
　bedtime 60
　colic 34, 59-60
CSF 117
curvature of the spine 98
cuts
　preventing 131
　what to do 137
cystic fibrosis 102-3

dark, fear of 61
day-stay surgery 127
daydreaming 153
deafness 79-81
death, child's response to 56-7
dehydration 105
delayed development 81-3
delinquency 151-2
demand feeding 32
dentist 48
depression, post-natal 16
developmental disability 81-3
diabetes
　adolescents 145
　young children 118-19

diarrhoea 105
digestive tract allergies 116
diphtheria immunisation 49-50
'dirty words' 63-4
disabled children see handicapped children
discipline 63
diseases see sickness
dislocation of the hip 97-8
disposable nappies 28
divorce 138
doctor
　advice 26
　choosing 16
　when to call 84-5
dogs 71
Down's syndrome 82
drowning 133
drugs
　see also medicines
　effect on embryo 18
　in milk 31-2
　use by adolescents 152-3
dummies 59

earache 87, 88
ears
　see also hearing
　infections 85-8
eating see feeding; meals
eczema 93
education see school
ejaculation of semen, first 146
electrical safety 132
embryo 18
emergency action 137, 155-7
　contacts 155
emotional development 44-7
encephalitis 100
epiglottitis 50
epilepsy 118
　in adolescence 145
erections 146
exercise 38, 39
external cardiac massage 156
eyes
　see also sight
　allergies 116
　at birth 19
　colour 89
　infections 88-90
　injuries 90

faces, baby recognising 43
failure to thrive 116-17
falls
　preventing 131
　what to do 137
fat children 38-40
fat deposits at birth 20
father
　at birth 54
　babies 22
　family without 139
　importance of 56
　single 139
fatigue 31
febrile convulsions 115
feeding

see also meals
baby 28-37
breast 28-30, 31-2
difficulties 34
formula 30-1
schedules 32-3
solids 34-5
weaning 34
feet 49
deformed 96
flat 97
fertilisation 17
fever 85, 98
convulsions 115
fighting 68
fire safety 134-5
fits see convulsions
flat feet 49, 97
flatulence 34
fluids
bottle-feeding 30
replacement 105
fluoride 30, 48
foetus 17-18
fontanelle 19
foods see feeding; meals
formula-feeding 30-1
foster parents 140
fungus infections 92, 94

garden safety 132
gastroenteritis 106-7
genes 18
genitals
disorders 108-10
growth 146
infant's interest in 66-7
German measles see rubella
glands, swollen 86-7
glasses (spectacles) 89
glue ear 88
goat's milk 30
gonorrhoea 108, 149-50
grandparents 23-4
helping working parents 141
'grasp reflex' 24
groin hernia 109
growing pains 95-6
gun safety 135
gurgling 25

haemophilus influenza type B 50, 117
hair at birth 20
handicapped children 78-83
adolescents 145
delayed development 81-3
physical 79-81
play 76-7
hands, baby's 24
hay fever 116
head
at birth 19
baby's 24
hydrocephalus 114
injuries 128
head-banging 59, 63
hearing 43
see also ears
deafness 79-81

heart disease 112-13
heat exhaustion 134
heat rashes 20, 91
height gain 42-3, 116
hepatitis B immunisation 50
hernia 109
HIBTiter 50, 117
hip dislocation 97-8
hitting children 63
HIV 149, 150
hives 95, 116
homosexuality 150
hospital
admission 125
advice from 26
child's questions 122-3
going home 129
living in 125-6
maternity, choosing 16
operations and anaesthetics 126-8
physiotherapy 128-9
pre-admission visiting 123
preparation for 121-5
visiting 125-6
what to take 123-4
Human Immunodeficiency Virus 149, 150
hydrocele 109
hydrocephalus 114
hydrotherapy 129
hypodermic needles 122, 125

identical twins 19
imagination 46
imitation 44, 70
immunisation 49-51, 98-101, 117
impetigo 93
incinerator safety 134-5
independence, growth of 55
individuality, growth of 55
infants see baby
infectious diseases 98-101
immunisation 49-51, 98-101, 117
ingested objects 132
inguinal hernia 109
inhaled objects 132
injuries
eye 90
sports 145
insect bites 95
insulin 118
intestinal problems 103-6
itchy eyes 90

jaundice at birth 20
JCA 96
jealousy 64
joint problems 95-8
juvenile chronic arthritis 96
juvenile delinquency 151-2

kidney
malformation 113
problems 107-8
kindergarten, meals for 37
knock-knees 49, 96

language see speaking
legs, bowed 49, 96
let-down reflex 29
leukemia 110
lips
at birth 20
blisters 91
cleft 113-14
long sight 89
loving your baby 22
lunch
baby's 35
for toddlers 37
weight reduction 39
lungs
allergies 116
malformation 113
lymph glands 87

malformations 111-14
genetic factors 18
malignant disease 110-11
masturbation
adolescents 146
infants 66
maternity hospital, choosing 16
meals
see also feeding
baby's 36-7
battles 41
eating non-food substances 63
for kindergarten and school 37
likes and dislikes 44
mother's, effect on breast-feeding 32
toddlers' 37
weight reduction 39
measles 99
immunisation 50
meconium 20
medicines 85
effect on breast-feeding 32
meningitis 50, 117-18
menstruation, commencement of 145-6
middle ear infections 87-8
milia 20
milk
allergy to 20-1
breast 28, 30
cow's 30
supply 32-3
weaning 34
milk rashes 20
'milk' teeth 47
moles 94
morning tea
for toddlers 37
weight reduction 39
mother
family without 139
relationship with baby 54-5
single 139
working 31, 141
Mothercraft support groups 26
motions see stools

mouth-to-mouth resuscitation 157
multiple births 19
mumps 99
immunisation 50
music 73

nail biting 66
nappies
buying 28
service 28
nappy rash 21, 92
navel hernia 109
needles, hypodermic 122, 125
nephritis 107
newborn baby 19-22
nipples, cracked 29, 34
nose
allergies 116
bleeds 86
infections 85-8
nursing see breast-feeding
nursing brassiere 31
Nursing Mothers Associations 26

obesity 38-9
operations 126-8
day-stay 127
explaining to child 121, 123
'oral gratification' 58
otitis externa 88
otitis media 87-8
outer ear infections 88
overweight 38
ovum 17

palate, cleft 113-14
pancreas, infamed 100
Parents Without Partners 139
pedestrian safety 135
penicillin 87
penis
circumcision 108-9
growth 146
periods, commencement of 145-6
pertussis see whooping cough
pets 71
physical handicaps 79-81
physical punishment 63
physiotherapy 128-9
pica 63
pimples 93-4, 146-7
placenta 17
plaster casts 128
play 72-3
development 45-6
handicapped children 76-77
material 68-9
purpose 68
safety 132
sick children 75-6
social development 70
with other children 70-1
playroom 69
pneumonia 101

poetry 73
poisoning
  preventing 131-2
  what to do 137
poliomyelitis vaccine 50
pool safety 134
'port wine stain' birthmark 94
posture, baby's 24
potty training 47
pregnancy
  emotions during 16
  teenage 149
premature babies 20
prickly heat rash 91
promises 45
psychological changes during adolescence 144
puberty 145-7
pubic hair at puberty 145, 146
puppets 73

rashes 91-2
  baby 20-1
  effect on surgery 127
reflexes 24, 29
resuscitation, mouth-to-mouth 157
right and wrong, concept of 44-5
ringworm 94
rivalry 64
road safety
  bicycles 135-6
  car travel 136
  pedestrians 135
rocking 59
'rooting reflex' 24, 29
roseola 101
roundworms 106
rubella 99
  effect on embryo 18
  immunisation 50
rumpus room 69

safe sex 149
safety
  accident prevention 130-6
  emergency action 137, 155-7
salt 35
sandpit 69
scalds
  preventing 131
  what to do 137
scalp 20
school
  deaf children 81
  for handicapped children 76
  meals for 37
scoliosis 98
seeing *see* sight
self-reliance, growth of 55
separated parents 138
separation of baby and mother 56
sex education 150
sexual behaviour
  adolescents 147-50
  young children 66-7
sharing 71
shoes 49
short sight 89
siblings *see* brothers and sisters
sickness
  adolescence 144-5
  bone and joint problems 95-8
  calling the doctor 84-5
  chest problems 101-3
  ear, nose and throat problems 85-8
  eye problems 88-90
  fever 85
  genital disorders 108-10
  infectious diseases 98-101
  intestinal problems 103-6
  kidney and bladder problems 107-8
  malformations 111-14
  malignant disease 110-11
  medicines 85
  play 75-6
  skin problems 90-5
SIDS 120
sight 43
  see also eyes
  blindness 81
  problems 89
sign language 80
single parents 139
sisters and brothers *see* brothers and sisters
skin
  see also rashes
  allergies 116
  at birth 19-21
  problems 90-5
skin cancers 134
skin contact 54
sleep disturbance 60-1
smiling 43
smoking 31-2
snake bites 95
snoring 87
social development 44-7
  importance of play 70
solid food, starting on 34-5
solo parents 139
soya bean milk 30
spanking 63
speaking
  bilingual 44
  deaf children 79
  development 43
  dirty 63-4
  problems 64-6
  to baby 25, 43
spectacles 89
speech *see* speaking
sperm 17
spider bites 95
spina bifida 114, 128
spine curvature 98
splash bath 69
splints 128
spoon feeding 35
sports injuries 145
squint 89
'startle reflex' 24
step families 139-40
stings 95
stomach aches 103
stools
  at birth 20
  constipation 103-4
  diarrhoea 105
  worms 106
stories 71
strabismus 89
strangers, fear of 44, 56
'strawberry' birthmark 94
streptococcal infections 107
stridor 86
stuttering 66
styes 89-90
'sucking reflex' 24, 29
sudden infant death syndrome 120
sugar 35, 38
'sun kicks' 92
sunblock 134
sunburn 134
surgery *see* operations
swallowed objects 132
'swear words' 63-4
'sweat test' for cystic fibrosis 102

talipes 96
talking *see* speaking
tantrums 46, 61-3
tea (beverage) 31
tea (meal)
  baby's 36
  for toddlers 37
  weight reduction 39
tear duct, blocked 89
teenagers *see* adolescents
teeth 47-9
  effect of dummies 59
  loose, and anaesthetics 128
teething 48
television 71
temper tantrums 46, 61-3
testicles
  growth 146
  hydrocele 109
  inflamed 99
  undescended 109-10
thin children 38-40
threadworms 106
threats 45
throat infections 85-8
thrush 92-3
thumb sucking 58
tick bites 95
tidiness 69
time, concept of 45
toddlers
books for 73-4
hospitalisation 121
jealousy 64
wakefulness 60-1
toilet training 47
tongue tie 65
tonsillitis 86-7
tonsils 87
toys 72-3
  as comforters 46
  box 69
  for sick children 76
  importance for social development 70
  material 68
traffic safety *see* road safety
travelling with children 52-3
triple antigen 49
truthfulness 46
tumours 110
twins 19

umbilical hernia 109
urine
  blood in 107-8
  infection 107

vaccination 49-51, 98-101, 117
vaginal discharge 108
venereal diseases 149-50
vernix 19
violence 63
viral infections 105, 115, 117
viruses 85-6, 98-101
vision *see* sight
vitamin supplements 30
vocabulary 43
voices
  baby's response to 43
  breaking 146
vomiting 34, 105

wading pool 69
wakefulness 60-1
warts 95
'water on the brain' 114
water safety 133-4
watering eyes 89
wax in the ears 88
weaning 34
weight
  gain 42-3, 116
  loss 38
  reduction 39
'wet dreams' 146
wheezing 102
whooping cough 100
  immunisation 49-50
wind 34
working parents 141-2
  breastfeeding 31
worms 106

X-rays, explaining to child 123

Your Child 160